Food-Based Natural Cosmetics

A Collection of Some Simple Home-Made Procedures

Agrihortico

CONTENTS

Natural Cosmetics: An Introduction 5

Apples As Natural Cosmetics 9

Almonds As Natural Cosmetics 16

Avocados As Natural Cosmetics 20

Bananas As Natural Cosmetics 24

Coconuts As Natural Cosmetics 28

Gooseberries as Cosmetics 35

Limes and Lemons as Natural Cosmetics 39

Oranges and Grapefruits As Natural Cosmetics 47

Papayas As Natural Cosmetics 50

Pomegranates As Natural Cosmetics 53

Walnuts As Natural Cosmetics 58

Beetroots As Cosmetics 61

Carrots As Cosmetics 65

Cucumbers As Natural Cosmetics 71

Onions as Natural Cosmetics 77

Tomatoes As Natural Cosmetics 79

Potatoes as Natural Cosmetics 83

Blackpepper as Natural Cosmetics 85

Cinnamon as Natural Cosmetics 87

Cloves as Natural Cosmetics 89

Garlic as Natural Cosmetics 91

Ginger Root As Natural Cosmetics 94

Turmeric As Natural Cosmetics 96

Curd and Yogurt as Natural Cosmetics 100

Ghee as a Natural Cosmetic 103

Milk and Milk Cream as Natural Cosmetics 105

Milk Powder As A Natural Cosmetic 109

Mustard Oil as a Natural Cosmetic 111

Olive Oil As A Natural Cosmetic 113

Pulses As A Natural Cosmetic 115

Rice Water as a Natural Cosmetic 119

Coffee As A Natural Cosmetic 121

Eggs as Natural Cosmetics 124

Honey and Beeswax as Natural Cosmetics 127

Sugar as a Natural Cosmetic 130

Tea as a Natural Cosmetic 133

Salt as Natural Cosmetics 136

Natural Cosmetics: An Introduction

Natural cosmetics are those cosmetics or beauty aids that can be prepared at home by using naturally available ingredients. In other words, natural cosmetics are those homemade remedies that we often use when we have some issues that spoil the way we look outward. For example, facial hair or acne on the face may spoil our attractive look and we tend to use some articles or products to improve our facial attractiveness. So cosmetics are nothing but the articles that we apply on our body for the cleansing and beautification purposes. It is often said that chemical cosmetics may have some side effects and allergic reactions if not used properly or if used in excess. Here comes the significance of natural cosmetics.

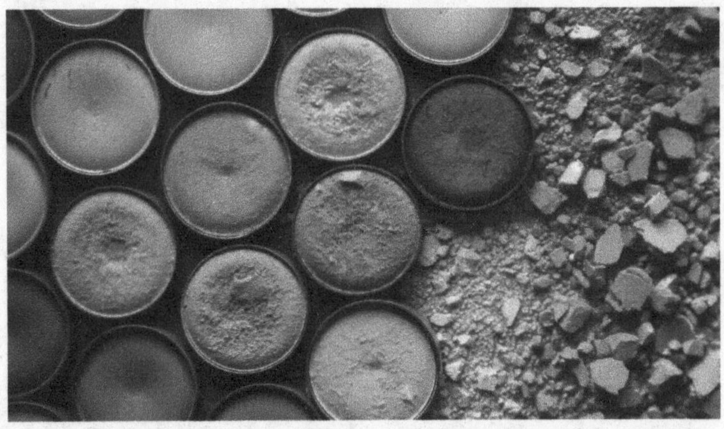

Natural cosmetics are nothing but those beauty products that are available to us in its pure, unadulterated forms. Most often, we use some of the foods that are easily available in our kitchens as natural cosmetics. So natural cosmetics are nothing but kitchen cosmetics. These kitchen cosmetics are natural and totally chemical free. Applying these cosmetics on face and skin provide us the natural glow that we have always desired for. Additionally, these kitchen cosmetics don't have any side effects. By using and applying homemade cosmetics regularly we can protect ourselves from chemical products available at the market. Chemical products not only have side effects but also its long term use makes our skin dull and dry. These natural home remedies not only save our money but also benefit our body in many other ways. In other words, home-made cosmetics are the best and the most affordable way to get that healthy, beautiful glowing face, skin, teeth and hair.

There are hundreds and hundreds of natural foods that can be used as natural cosmetics or kitchen cosmetics or home-made cosmetics. Out of these the most beneficial and affordable foods are as listed below:

1. Turmeric: Fresh turmeric and turmeric powder
2. Lemons and limes: Juice and zest or rind of the limes and lemons
3. Oranges: Mainly dried and powdered peel of the oranges
4. Coconut Oil: Pure coconut oil has cooling and soothing effect on human body. Its regular use

removes scar marks and dead skin cells from body.

5. Olive Oil: Lots of medicinal properties are attributed to olive oil. Regular use of olive oil improves body's blood circulation.
6. Dairy Products: Milk, Milk Cream etc
7. Sugar: Adding sugar granules in face masks and massage creams cleanses and nourishes the body.
8. Coffee and Tea: These hot beverages can also play some role in improving our beauty.
9. Eggs: Beaten egg white can be used as a skin-tightening face mask.
10. Honey: Pure honey is known for its anti-ageing benefits.
11. Rice Water: This is a home-made natural hair-conditioner that can be used for healthy growth of the hair.
12. Bengal Gram: In fact, bengal gram powder is one of the best ingredients that can be added to any face mask preparations because of its skin-tightening properties.
13. Greengram: Greengram powder is a natural product that can e used for promoting good hair growth.

In addition to the above-mentioned products, there are a large varieties of fruits and nuts, vegetables, spices and condiments, cereals and millets, pulses, etc. that are always present in our kitchens, can be used in various ways to improve our attractiveness and skin health. By using these home remedies you can easily deal with various skin problems such as acne, dark spots, blemishes, dark circles, dry skin, oily skin etc and hair problems such as dandruff, dry scalp and hair fall.

Fruits and nuts, vegetables and other foods such as cereals and millets, pulses etc are very popular among all of us as healthy foods and therefore, these foods are always present in our kitchens. Isn't it interesting to know that these foods such as vegetables, fruits and nuts can be used in other ways also? Like using them as ingredients for making natural cosmetics. However, a word of caution here. ***Not all vegetables, fruits and nuts and other types of foods such as millets, pulses etc are suitable for cosmetic preparations***.

A detailed account of those foods that can be used as beauty aids is given in the following chapters.

Apples As Natural Cosmetics

All of us have heard of this proverb that says, *"An apple a day, keeps the doctor away"*. An apple is not only helpful for our health but it is also very beneficial for our skin also. It contains lots of nutrients which can make our skin healthy. An apple helps to reduce the wrinkles. Apples also protect our skin from UV rays and help to build healthy hair and eyes. In small amount it also helps in skin-brightening. So let us rephrase the proverb, ***"An apple a day, I am young forever."***

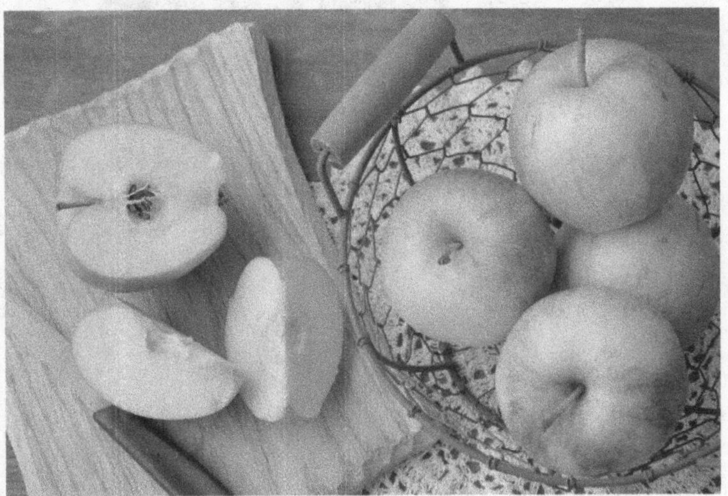

Apples for Weight Management: Eating fresh apples or apple-based diet regularly is considered as a major step in all weigh management programs. Apple helps in losing extra body weight and is considered as one of the best foods for weight loss.

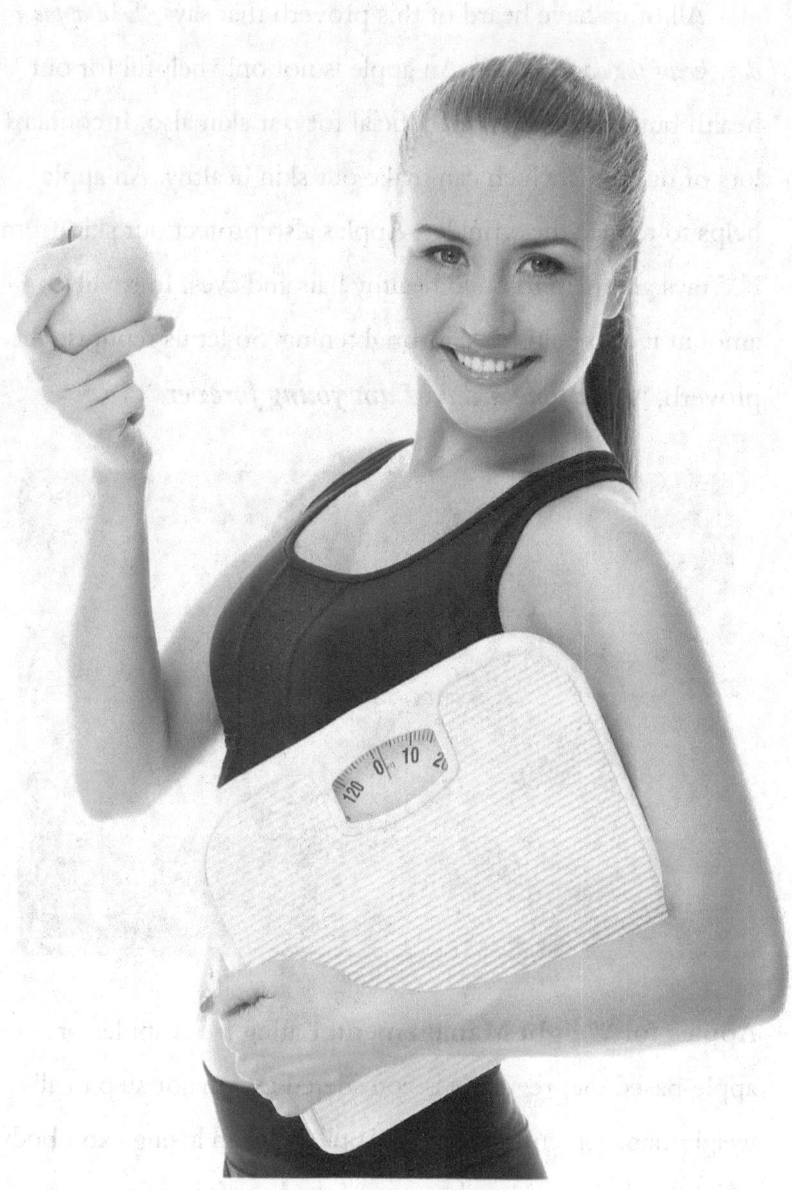

Now let us have a deep insight into the process and method of apple-based natural cosmetic preparations.

Apple for Teeth: Use good quality crunchy apples for oral health. By biting and chewing an apple, the production of saliva in the mouth gets reduced and as a result, bacterial activity in the mouth is minimized. Mouth remains fresh for hours and bad odor in the mouth is completely eliminated. Eating an apple a day helps you get white, shiny and healthy teeth.

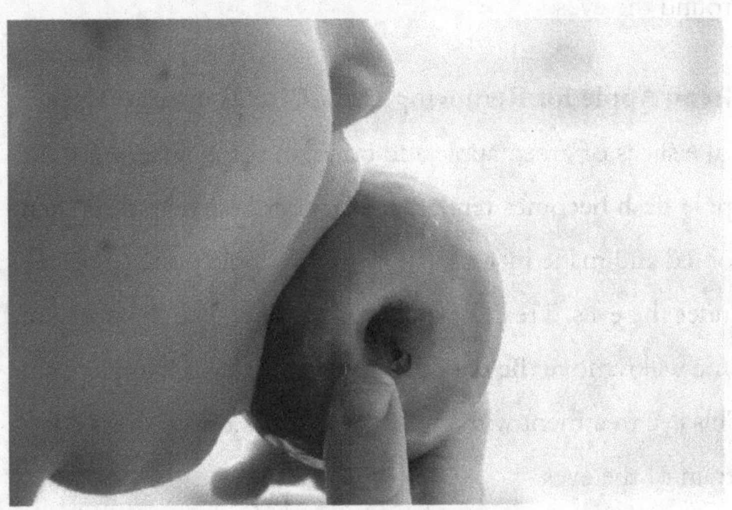

Apple Cider Vinegar for Dandruff: Mix ¼ cup of apple cider vinegar into ¼ cup of water. Take an empty spray bottle and fill it with this mixture. Spray this on your hair and scalp before going to bed. Repeat this process 3-4 times in a week regularly for few weeks. Your dandruff is gone in no time.

Apple Slices for Removing Eye Infections: Take an unripe apple and cut it into few thick long slices. Now roast it on a fire. Let it cool down. When it is in normal room temperature, apply it on your eyes. This can help you protect your eyes from any kind of eye infections and helps treat swelling of eyes and also redness of eyes.

Apple Slices for Removing Dark Circles Around Eyes: Slices of fresh apple is also good for eyes. Keeping thin slices of fresh apple under the eyes helps you get rid of dark circles around the eyes.

Green Apple for Removing Dark Circles around Eyes: Take slices of green apple and boil it in some water until the apple flesh becomes tender. This tender boiled apple is then cooled and made into a paste. Use this apple paste to place under the eyes. Treating your eyes regularly like this for some time will remove the dark patches of your eyes completely. This eye treatment with apple paste also reduces stress and strain of the eyes.

Apple for Skin Hydration: Take fresh apples. Wash it thoroughly. Now cut it into thin slices and cover your face with these slices. Wait until the slices become dry (wait almost for 20-25 minutes). Remove the slices when it is completely dried. This treatment leaves your skin hydrated and healthy.

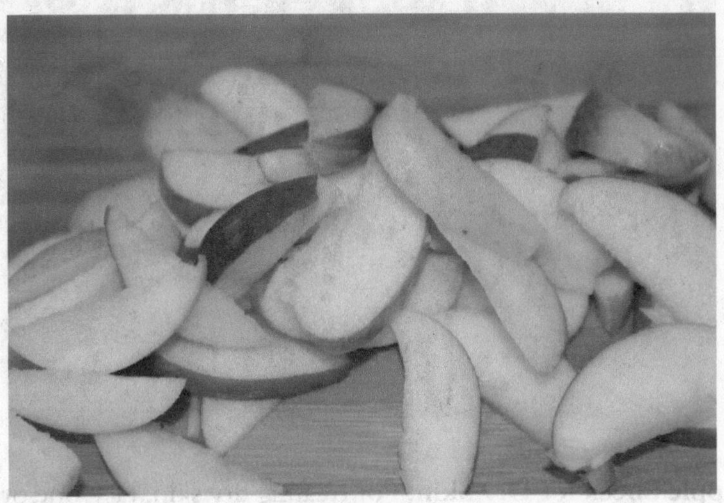

Apple for Making Natural Face Mask: First of all refrigerate thin slices of an apple. After few hours, when apple slices are chilled, take it out, mash it and add small amount of milk cream. Mix all the ingredients well and make a paste. Apply the paste on your face. Leave it for 10 minutes and then rinse off with cold water. Use this beauty treatment regularly for a few days. It helps you get rid of facial acne, blemishes and dark spots quickly.

Apple Juice as a Natural Skin Toner: You can use freshly made apple juice as a natural toner. Use a cotton ball to apply this toner on your face. Apply it regularly for glowing facial skin.

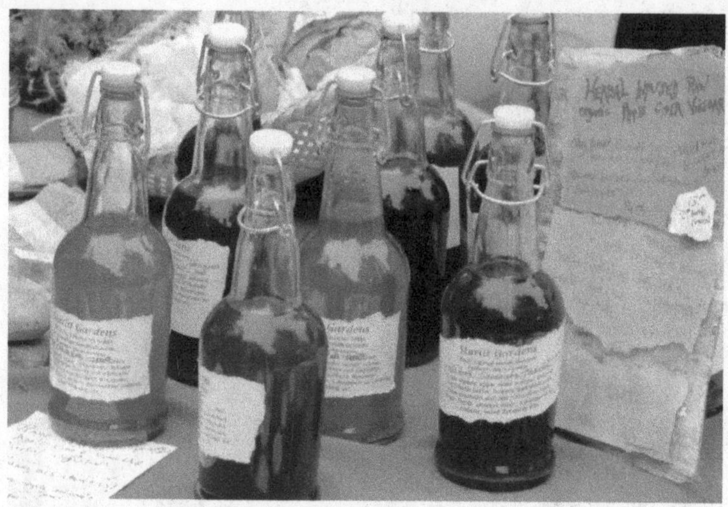

Apple Slices for Dry Skin: For treating dry skin, take one or two slices of an apple and rub it on your face until it dries up. Then wash your face with cold water. This helps you reduce the dryness of skin leaving your skin nourishing and hydrating.

Apple for Making Moisturizer: For making apple moisturizer, take an apple, peel the outer layer and remove the inner hard part and make a puree. Now add one spoonful each of honey and milk cream. Mix all the ingredients well and make a paste. Use this paste as a moisturizer regularly to make your skin soft and smooth.

Apple Cider Vinegar for Healing Sunburn: Take ½ cup of apple cider vinegar; add 4 cups of water into it. Mix the ingredients well and make a solution. Take a clean white muslin cloth and dip it in the solution. Apply this solution gently on sunburned skin. Massage for a while. Repeat this procedure several times in a day for days until the condition improves.

Apple Cider Vinegar for Smelly Feet: Take one bowl of apple cider vinegar and add 4 bowls of water into it to make a solution. Now soak your feet in the solution for 15 minutes. Then rinse and dry your feet. This will help you remove the bad smell and bacteria from your feet.

Apple Cider Vinegar as a Nail Cleanser: Take equal quantities of apple cider vinegar and water into a bowl and soak your fingernails into it for at least 20 minutes. Then rinse off. Use it twice a day to make your nail nice and bright.

Almonds As Natural Cosmetics

Almond is a very popular nut which is consumed worldwide for its various health benefits. These nuts are a fantastic source of antioxidants and are high in Vitamin E also. Almonds can reduce hunger and promote weight loss. Almonds are very useful for people with diabetes as it helps control the blood sugar. Eating almonds not only sharpens our mind but also helps us with a healthy and glowing skin.

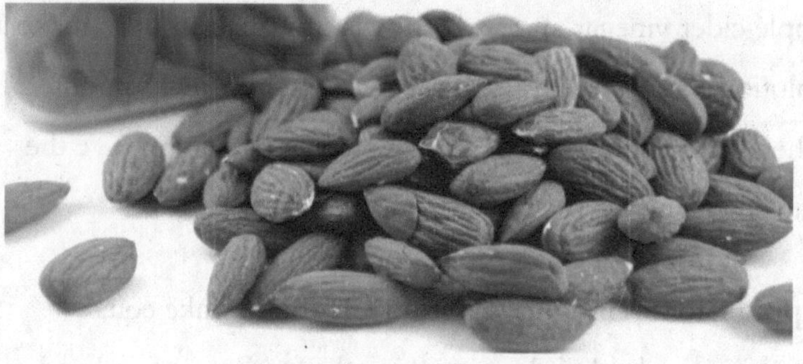

Almonds for Preventing Premature Ageing: Soak 6-7 almonds overnight and peel their skins off in the morning. Then grind the peeled almonds into a smooth paste. Add 5-6 drops of coconut milk into the almond paste. Mix well and apply this paste on your face for 15 minutes and wash it off with cold water. This almond-based cosmetic preparation helps you prevent wrinkles, sagging skin and age spots.

Almond Oil for Eyes: Almond oil is very effective for puffy eyes, dark circles and eye wrinkles. It improves your eyesight and provides relief from eye stress. This oil is beneficial for the people who are working on the computer all day long. You only have to do a gentle oil massage on eyelids. Regular application of almond oil on eyes also helps you get thick and long eyelashes.

Almond Oil for Relaxation: You can even use almond oil as a body massage oil. Massage your body thoroughly with this oil. Almond oil massage helps you feel relaxed and refreshed and also improves the blood circulation throughout the body.

Almond Oil as a Natural Makeup Remover: Almond oil is a great substitute to all the chemical makeup-removers.

Almond Oil Promotes Hair Growth: Massaging your hair with almond oil at least thrice a week can help to promote your hair growth. This hair treatment also makes your hair strong, shiny and soft. It also ensures the growth of silky and non-frizzy hair and delays greying of hair too.

Almonds for Curing Dandruff: Intake of almonds on regular basis can help to prevent dandruff and inflammation. Eating almonds not only sharpens your brain but it also moisturizes and nourishes your scalps and promotes healthy hair growth.

Almond Oil for Treating Acne: For treating your acne, mix one tablespoon of almond oil with one tablespoon of lemon juice. Apply this solution on the face with the help of a cotton pad every day till acne and acne scars are diminished. .

Almond Oil for Dry Skin: In a small spray bottle, add two tablespoons of almond oil and one tablespoon of rose water. Shake it and mix the ingredients well. Spray it on your face as a toner before applying any moisturizer. Use this spray everyday for better results. Store this home-made natural toner in the refrigerator for later use.

Almond Oil for Soft Lips: If you use almond oil daily on your lips as a lip balm, it will make your lips naturally soft and pink. Apply almond oil before going to bed every day.

Almond Oil for Pink/Red Lips: Take a beetroot and cut it into small pieces and dry it in the sun. These sun-dried beetroot pieces are then made into a smooth powder by grinding it. Mix one pinch of this beetroot powder with one tablespoon of almond oil to make a thick paste. Apply this thick paste on the lips and wait for 10 minutes. After 10 minutes, wash it off with lukewarm water. Repeat this process once in a day for a few days for better results.

Almond Oil for Cracked Heels: For curing cracked heels, take equal amounts of almond oil and rose water in a bowl and shake well to mix the ingredients. Rub this mixture on your feet every day before you go to bed. Rinse off with lukewarm water next morning. Repeat this process for a few weeks for complete cure.

Almond Oil for Clearing Sun-Tanning: Take a bowl and

add one tablespoon of bengal gram flour in it. Now add one tablespoon each of lemon juice and almond oil. Mix the ingredients well to form a thick paste. Now apply this mixture on sun-tanned parts of the body. Wait for 15 minutes and then wash it off with lukewarm water. Repeat the process until your sun-tanning goes away.

Almond Oil for Reducing Dark Circles: Dip a cotton pad in almond oil and apply it all over the delicate skin of the eyes. This will reduce the puffiness under your eyes and also help in getting rid of the dark circles.

Almond Oil for Nails: For longer, stronger nails, you can always rely on almond oil. When you clip your nails or remove your nail paint, apply some almond oil on your cuticles. Doing this once every day will improve the growth and health of your nails. It's perfect for healing brittle and chipped nails also.

Avocados As Natural Cosmetics

The stone fruit-avocado is a very healthy and nutrient-rich fruit. They contain more potassium than that of bananas. Eating avocados can help lower cholesterol levels. Avocados also keep your eyes healthy. Avocado helps you to get moisturized and hydrated skin. Avocados have anti-inflammatory and anti-ageing properties as well.

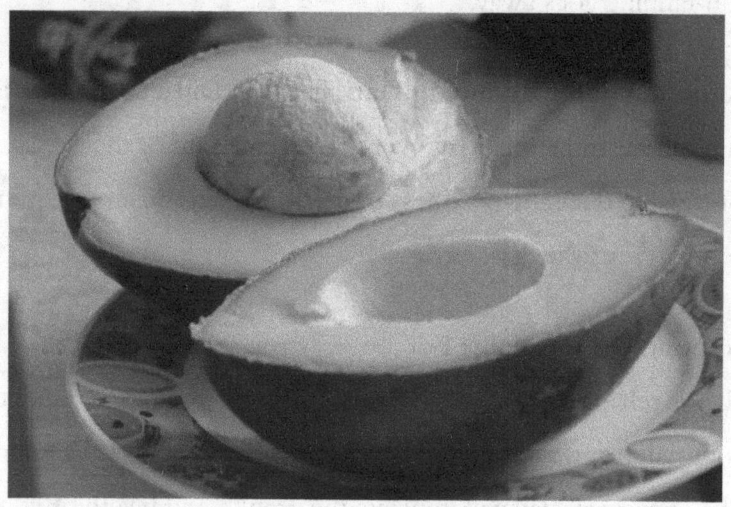

Avocados for Treating Acne: Scoop out inner part (only flesh) of an avocado and mash it well. Now add one tablespoon of honey to it and mix both the ingredients well to make a paste. Apply this avocado mask on your face, wait for 15 minutes and then rinse off with cold water. Apply avocado facial mask thrice a week for better results.

Avocados for Removing Dead Skin Cells: Mash one half of an avocado (only flesh) in a bowl and add one spoonful of oatmeal in it. Mix the ingredients well to make a thick facial mask. Apply this mask on your face and then leave it on for 15 minutes before rinsing off with cold water. This beauty treatment will clear your skin by removing all dead cells from the skin.

Avocado-Apricot Facial Mask for Removing Dead Skin Cells: Take an avocado and an apricot. Blend both the fruits well to make a thick paste. Put it on your face as a mask. Sit for 30 minutes and then wash your face with cold water. This mask can help exfoliate dead skin cells and also tighten the facial skin. This beauty treatment helps balance skin tone as well.

Avocado for Treating Dry Skin: Take an avocado and cut it into two halves. Scoop out the inner flesh and mash it properly. Now add one spoonful of yogurt and ½ spoonful of honey. Mix all the ingredients well to make a paste. Apply this paste on the face as a mask. Wait for 15-20 minutes and rinse off with cold water. Do this 2-3 times a week to achieve the desired results very quickly.

Avocado Oil for Treating Dandruff: For treating dandruff problem, take hot avocado oil and gently apply it on your hair scalp. Use it as a hot oil mask whenever you want to oil your hair. This treatment will help reduce dandruff occurrence on scalp and also keep your scalp healthy always.

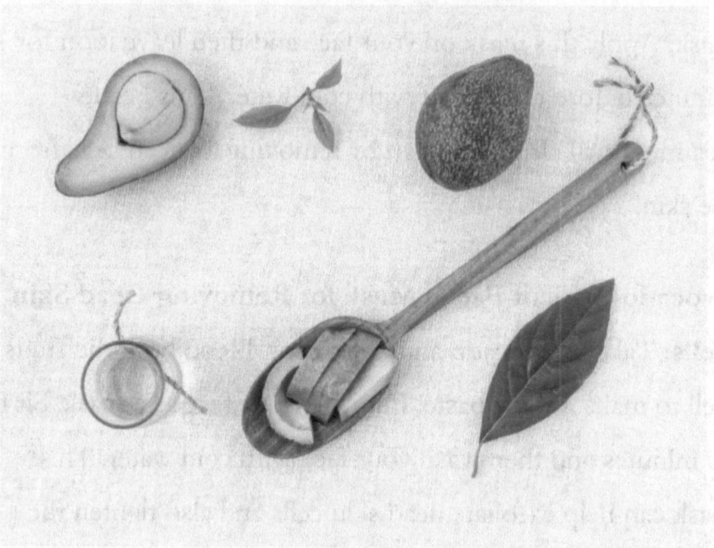

Avocado Pulp as a Facial Moisturizer: Take the inner flesh of an avocado and apply gently on your face. Leave it for 15 minutes. Then rinse off with cold water. This will help you get your facial skin nourished and moisturized.

Avocado and Honey Mask as a Facial Toner: Take a ¼ part of an avocado and one spoonful of honey and one spoonful of yogurt. Mix these ingredients well to make a paste. Apply it on your face as a mask and leave the mask on for 10-15 minutes. Then rinse off with cold water. This beauty treatment is very effective to treat acne.

Avocado Oil as a Bath Oil: Use 2-3 spoonful of avocado oil to the bath water. Taking bath in this water will make your whole body feel soft.

Avocado Slices for Removing Blackheads: For treating blackheads on your face, take a few slices of a fresh avocado. Rub these slices on your face in circular motion for a few minutes. This treatment will remove the blackheads and restore the skin to its natural glow.

Avocado for Anti-Ageing: Take one ripe avocado and one spoonful of coconut oil. Mix the ingredients well to make a paste. Apply this paste on your face as a facial mask. Wait for 10 minutes and then wash off with cold water. Use this thrice a week. This beauty treatment is effective for eliminating age spots and wrinkles on the face.

Avocado for Removing Excess Skin Oil: Scoop out inner flesh of an avocado and add one beaten egg and one spoonful of lemon juice into it. Mix these ingredients well to make a paste. Apply thick layer of this paste as a mask on your face and wait for 20-25 minutes. Then wash it off with cold water.

Note: Instead of lemon juice you can use pulp of a small banana.

Bananas As Natural Cosmetics

Banana is a very popular nutritious fruit which is available across the world. Banana is an instant energy booster fruit. Banana helps maintain a healthy nervous system; lower cholesterol level and enhances gut health. Banana fruit can be used for cosmetic purposes also such as for making banana face masks, banana-based natural skin moisturizer and skin cream.

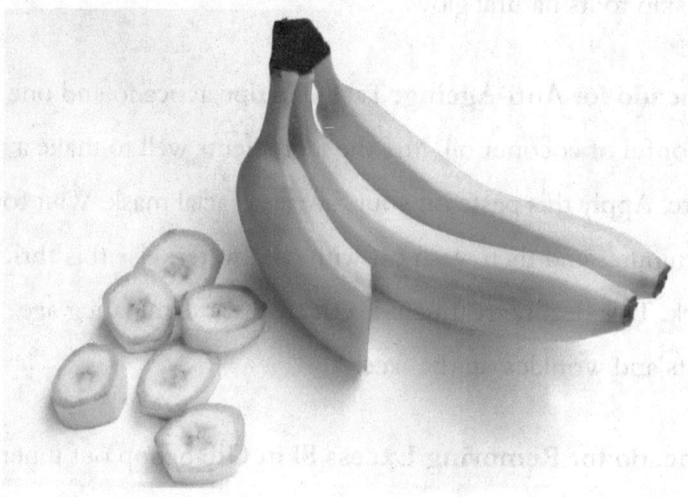

Banana as a Skin Moisturizer: Take a ripe banana and mash it properly. Apply it on your face. Then wait for 20-25 minutes before washing it off with cold water. This beauty treatment will instantly moisturize your facial skin.

Banana as a Hair Conditioner: Take one peeled ripe banana in a bowl and mash it thoroughly to make a paste. Then add ½ spoonful of honey and mix it well. Your banana-based hair conditioner is ready. Use it just like any other hair conditioners.

Banana for Curing Cracked Heels and Dry Feet: Take a ripe banana and mash it to make a paste. Apply this paste on feet and leave it for half an hour. After that wash your feet with lukewarm water. Repeat the process until you get soft feet.

Banana Mask for Treating Hair Fall: Take 3-4 ripe peeled bananas and pulp from 2-3 leaves of aloe vera plant. Put aloe vera pulp and peeled bananas in a blender and blend it until it becomes a thick paste. Use this paste as a hair mask on your hair and leave it for two to three hours. After that wash your hair with shampoo and lukewarm water. Repeat the process for a few days to get the better results.

Banana Peel for Curing Tired and Puffy Eyes: Eat your banana but don't throw its peel away. Banana peel is very helpful to reduce puffy eyes. Make small circular pieces of banana peel and place it on your eyes. Leave it on for half an hour. After half an hour wash your eyes with cold water. This treatment will definitely reduce the puffiness of eyes.

Banana Peel for Treating Facial Acne: Make small circular pieces of banana peel and rub it on your facial acne for a few minutes. After that wash your face with cold water. Do it thrice a day. This will help reduce the growth and redness of acne.

Banana Peel for White Teeth: Make small circular pieces of banana peel and rub it on your teeth for a few minutes. Then leave it for 10 minutes. Now brush your teeth with your favorite toothpaste. Do it morning and evening every day for a few days for better results.

Banana Mask for Treating Oily Face: Take one thoroughly mashed banana, one spoonful of honey and ½ spoonful of lemon. Mix all the ingredients well to make a paste. Now apply this paste as a face mask and leave it on for 10-15 minutes before washing it off with cold water. This beauty treatment may be done twice or thrice a week for better results.

Banana for Clearing Dark Spots on Face: Using a mashed banana on your face twice a week will help you clear dark spots on the face.

Banana for Brighter and Glowing Skin: Take one thoroughly mashed banana, one spoonful of raw milk, one spoonful of honey and some drops of rose water. Mix all the ingredients well to make a paste. Apply it on your face. Leave it for 15 minutes. Wash your face with water. This beauty treatment will help you get brighter and glowing skin.

Banana for Clearing Wrinkles: Take one thoroughly mashed banana, one spoonful of orange juice and one spoonful of plain yogurt. Apply it on your face and let it sit there for 15-20 minutes. After that wash it off with cold water. This beauty treatment reduces the wrinkles and fine lines on the face.

Banana Mask for Hair Growth: Take two thoroughly mashed bananas and one beaten egg. Mix the ingredients well until the mixture gets a good consistency. Now apply it on your hair and leave it for 15 minutes. After that rinse off your hair with lukewarm water. Using this beauty treatment regularly will help you grow long and healthy hair.

Banana Mask for Silky and Dandruff-Free Hair: Take two thoroughly mashed bananas and one spoonful of coconut oil. Mix it well. Apply it on your hair and wait for 15 minutes. Then rinse off your hair with lukewarm water. This beauty treatment can be done regularly until the dandruff goes away.

Coconuts As Natural Cosmetics

Coconut is the fruit of the coconut palm tree and it is considered as a nutritious fruit that helps in improving bone health. Consuming coconut flesh regularly may have several health benefits such as weight loss, improved heart health, proper digestion, improved brain health, control of blood sugar levels and improved immunity. Tender coconut water is considered as a healthy and nutritious natural drink.

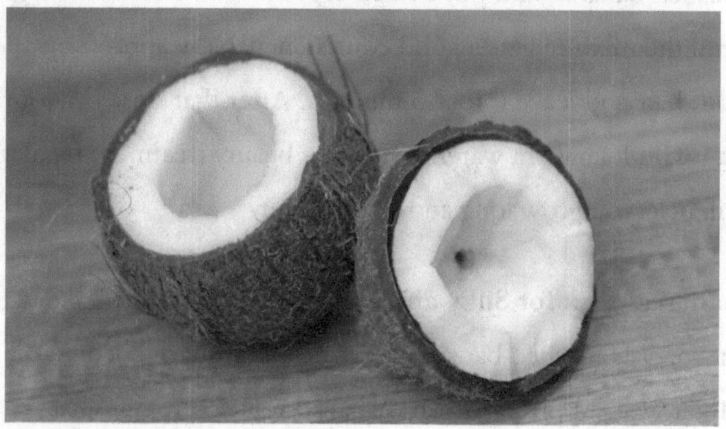

Coconut Oil as a Breath Freshener: Gargling with pure coconut oil for 20 minutes helps clear up germs in the mouth and it also leads to fresher breath, white teeth and healthy gums.

Coconut Oil as a Remedy for Lice Infestation: First of all, rinse off your hair with a cup of apple cider vinegar. Let the hair dry. After that, apply coconut oil thoroughly on your head and leave it for 24 hours. Now brush your hair with a fine comb to collect the dead lice. After removing the dead lice, wash the hair off with a shampoo and conditioner.

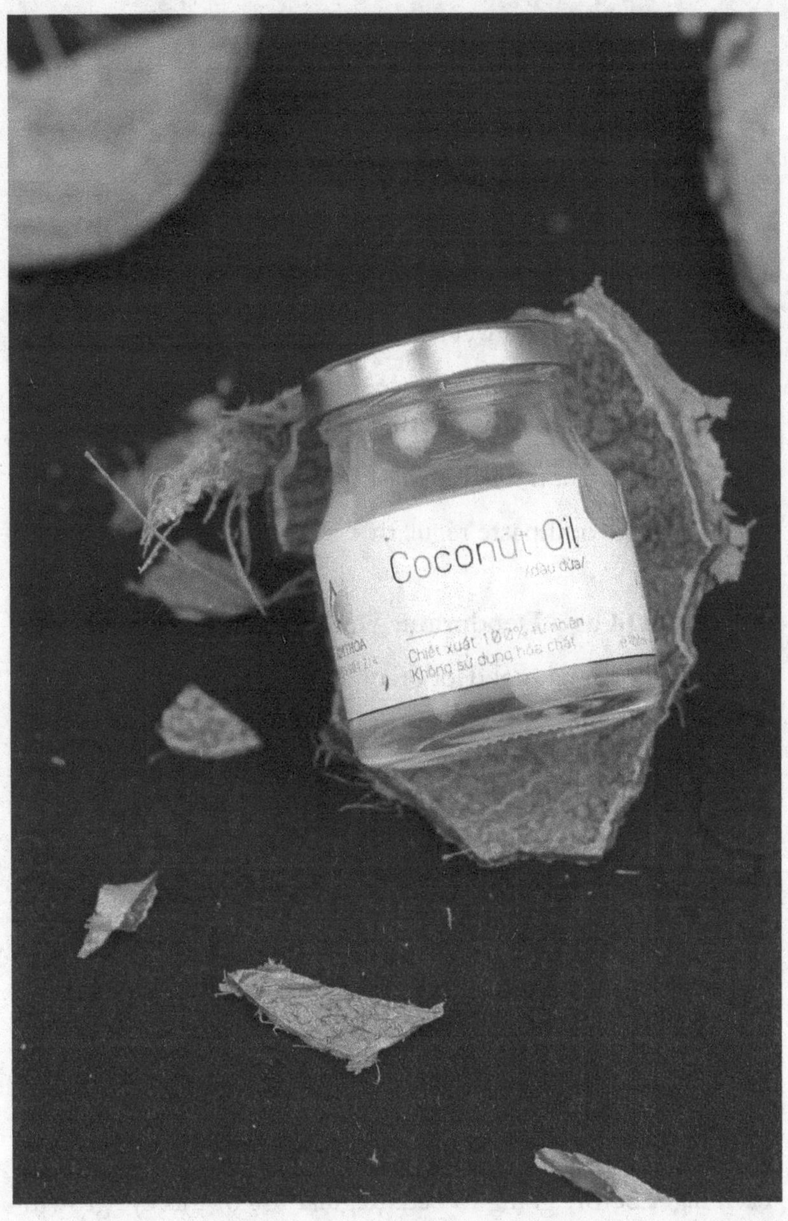

Coconut Oil as a Body Moisturizer: Coconut oil is a natural body moisturizer. Regular use of coconut oil as a moisturizer is advised during summer season due to its cooling and hydrating effect on body.

Coconut Oil as a Lip Balm: Coconut oil is the best way to get rid of chapped lips.

Coconut Oil as an Eye Cream: Coconut oil can be used as an under eye cream as well.

Coconut Oil for White Teeth: Take one tablespoon of coconut oil and add one pinch of baking soda. Mix it well and then use it as toothpaste regularly for getting white teeth.

Coconut Oil as a Deodorant: You can use coconut oil to make your own natural deodorant at home. Take one tablespoon of coconut oil and add one pinch each of arrowroot powder, corn starch, and baking soda. Mix all the ingredients well. Finally add fragrant oil (such as tea tree oil and pepper mint oil) for an odor fix. Natural deodorant is ready.

Coconut Oil as Eyelash Growth Serum: Mix a tablespoon of coconut oil with one drop of lemon essential oil and one drop of lavender oil. Mix and apply the same to your eye lashes each night before going to bed. Regular use of this eye growth serum results in thick and long eyelash growth.

Coconut Water for Curing Dry Skin: Mix coconut water with turmeric powder until you get a fine paste. Now add a few drops of coconut oil into this paste. Apply this paste to your face as a mask and let it sit there for 10 minutes. Then wash it off with cold water. This face mask will cure your dry skin immediately.

Coconut Water for Treating Acne: Washing your face with coconut water before going to bed regularly will decrease the acne occurrence on your face.

Coconut Water as a Skin Toner: Soak a washed cloth in coconut water. Scrub this cloth all over your skin. Go to bed with coconut water still in place. You will get smoother and more even skin. This also may help reduce signs of aging.

Coconut Water for Treating Dry Scalp: If you have dry scalp and dandruff, then simply wash the scalp with coconut water regularly. This can help moisturize the scalp and reduce the presence of dandruff.

Coconut Scrub Cream for Cleansing and Nourishing Body: A coconut scrub cream may be made with the inner flesh of the coconut. Regular use of this scrub cream will cleanse and nourish your body perfectly.

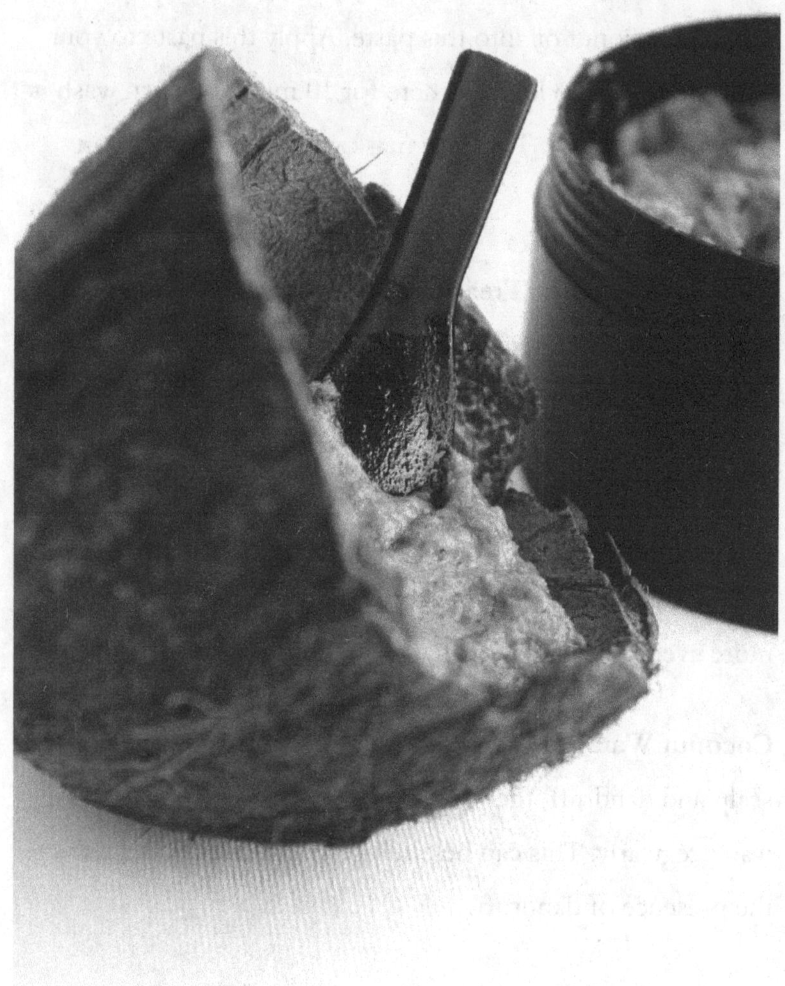

Coconut Water as a Refreshing Soft Drink: Drinking coconut water helps you keep energetic and fresh.

Coconut Water as a Makeup Remover: You can apply coconut water using cotton pad to remove your makeup.

Coconut Milk for Dry Hair: Coconut milk can be used as scalp tonic for dry, itchy and irritated scalp. You can get a good nourishing effect if you do a head massage with coconut milk for half an hour. After the massage, cover your head with a hot towel for some time for better results.

Coconut Milk for Hair Growth: Apply coconut milk on your hair and leave it on 20 minutes before shampooing your hair as usual. This hair treatment will promote good hair growth.

Coconut Milk for Hair Conditioning: Take equal amounts of coconut milk and your favorite shampoo. Mix both the ingredients well to make a hair conditioner. Apply it on your hair regularly for better results.

Coconut Milk as a Makeup Remover: To remove your makeup, make a mixture by adding 2 spoonful of olive oil and one spoonful of coconut milk. Rub this mixture gently on your face by using a cotton pad to remove your make up.

Coconut Milk as a Facial Scrub: You can even use coconut milk as a face scrub for gentle exfoliation. For making a coconut milk-based face scrub, just soak some oats in coconut milk for 10 minutes. Mash the mixture thoroughly. Use this mixture as a scrubber on face on regular basis for better results.

Coconut Milk for Treating Sunburns: Application of coconut milk over sun-burnt skin helps in fast healing. It helps healing by cooling the skin and reducing the pain, swelling and redness.

Coconut Milk for Moisturizing Skin: You can rub coconut milk on your skin directly for 20-30 minutes to reduce dryness and promote healthy glowing skin.

Coconut Milk for Bath Water: You can add equal quantities of coconut milk and rose water to your bath water for all kinds of beauty benefits.

Gooseberries as Cosmetics

Indian gooseberry or Amla is a sour and nutritious fruit which is known for its high Vitamin C content. Gooseberry helps in boosting our immune system, in reducing signs of aging, and also helpful in treating throat infections. Gooseberries are known for its ability to reduce blood sugar levels and thus managing the diabetes effectively. It also improves heart health.

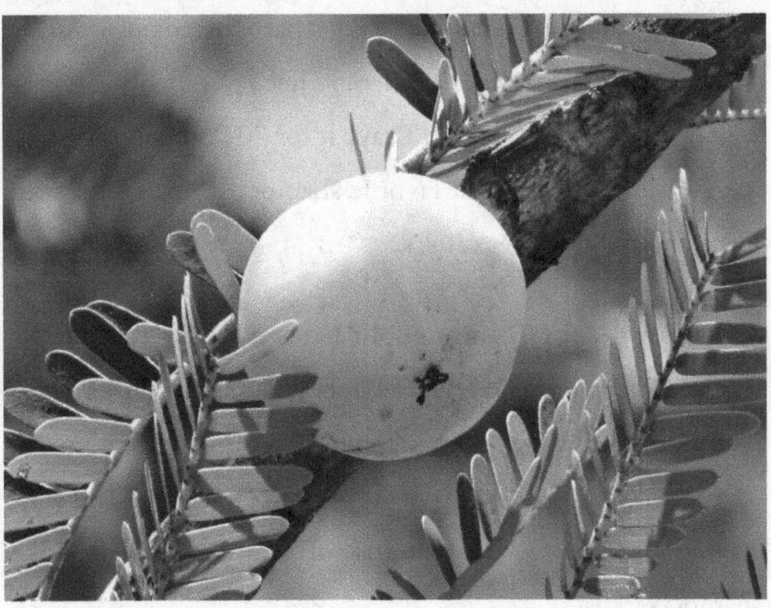

From time immemorial, gooseberries are used as traditional Ayurvedic medicines for improving skin and scalp health. Gooseberry hair oil or Amla oil is recommended in these traditional medicines as an effective remedy for headaches. Amla hair oil is known as effective oil for the growth of thick and healthy hair. By consuming gooseberries regularly we can reap both the health and the cosmetic benefits of these fruits.

Amla Powder for Smooth and Clean Skin: Take amla powder and add one spoonful each of yogurt and honey into it. Mix the ingredients well to make a paste and apply this paste as a mask on your face. Let it dry and then wash it with cold water. This mask will give you smooth and clean skin. This beauty treatment will leave your skin glowing and hydrated too.

Amla Powder for Hair Fall: Make a paste by mixing one small cup of amla powder and lemon juice of one big lemon in water. Apply it on your hair. Leave it for 20-25 minutes and then wash it off with your favorite shampoo. Do this treatment twice a week for better results.

Amla Powder for Treating Split Ends of Hair: Take one small cup each of henna powder and amla powder in a bowl. Now add plain yogurt or curd to it. Mix all the ingredients well to make a smooth paste. Apply this paste on wet hair and leave it on for 1-2 hours. After that rinse off your hair with a mild shampoo.

Amla Powder for Reducing Face Oil: Make a paste of two tablespoons of amla powder in rose water. Apply it on the face and leave for 15-20 minutes and then wash it off with water. Repeat this treatment twice a week for better results.

Amla Powder for Frizzy and Dry Hair: Take two beaten eggs in a bowl and add half a cup of amla powder. Mix the ingredients well to make a paste. Now apply this paste on your hair scalp. Wait for one or two hours. Then wash off with a mild shampoo. Do this once a week for better results.

Amla Oil for Hair Care: Applying amla oil to the roots of your hair improves hair growth and color. It helps reduce the chances of hair loss and baldness. Massaging hair with amla oil strengthens the roots, maintains color and improves luster. It also treats dandruff and dryness of scalp.

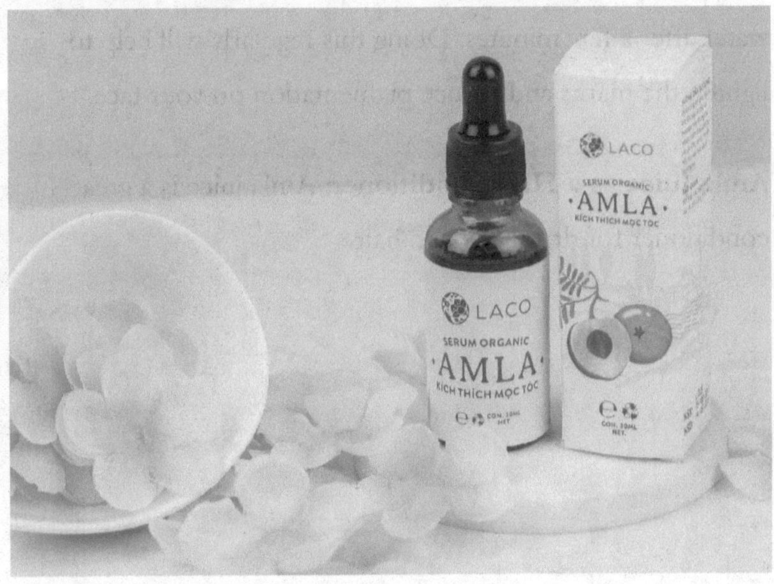

Amla Juice for Scalp Cleaner: Amla juice is great for cleansing the scalp. It helps to nourish the scalp and makes your hair shiny. It helps to protect our hair from various hair damages caused due to dust, pollution, smoke etc.

Amla Juice for Reducing Pigmentation: Apply amla juice on your face by using a cotton ball and then rinse it off with water after a few minutes. Doing this regularly will help to lighten the marks and reduce pigmentation on your face.

Amla Juice as a Hair Conditioner: Amla juice is a great conditioner for dry and rough hair.

Limes and Lemons as Natural Cosmetics

Lemons are high in Vitamin C content which is beneficial for heart health, weight management and digestive health. Consuming lemon juice in the morning in empty stomach helps to reduce belly fat. Lemons help in soothing a sore throat and an upset stomach. Lemon fruits have lots of cosmetic benefits too.

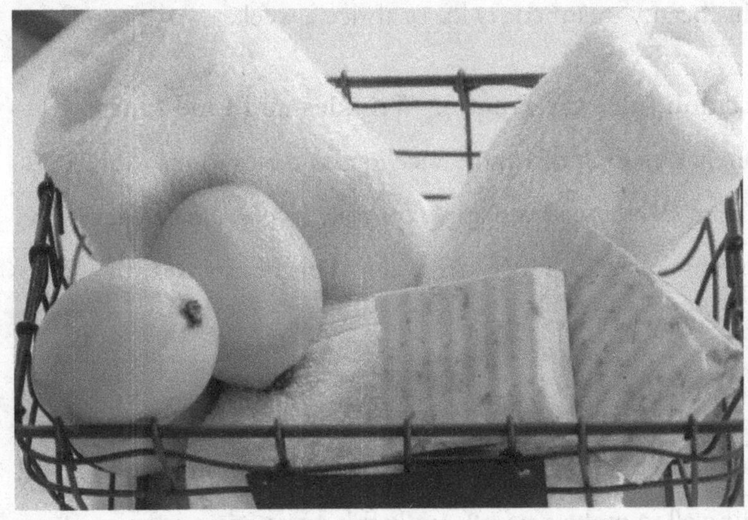

Lemon Juice for Dark Spots: Mix half a spoon of lemon juice in two spoonful of plain yogurt. Then add a few drops of rose water. Mix all the ingredients well to form a paste and apply the paste on your face evenly. After 20 minutes, wash it off with cold water and apply some moisturizer. This beauty treatment will help you to get rid of dark spots and blemishes from your facial skin.

Lemon Juice for Removing Excess Oil and Acne from Face: Take one spoonful of honey, ¼ spoon of turmeric powder and ½ spoon of lemon juice. Mix them well and apply on your face. Wait for 15 minutes and rinse off with water. Use this beauty treatment twice or thrice a week.

Lemon Juice for Treating Wrinkles and Fine Lines: Add one tablespoon of lemon juice in two tablespoons of milk cream. Mix it well and apply on your face as a face pack. After 10 minutes wash it off with water. This beauty treatment helps to reduce wrinkles and fine lines.

Lemon Juice for Hair Growth: Take fresh gel from one aloe vera leaf in a bowl. Add one spoonful of lemon juice to it and stir well to make a paste. Apply this paste on your hair and scalp. Wait for half an hour and rinse it off with a mild shampoo. Do this treatment once a week to reduce your hair fall. This treatment also promotes healthy hair growth.

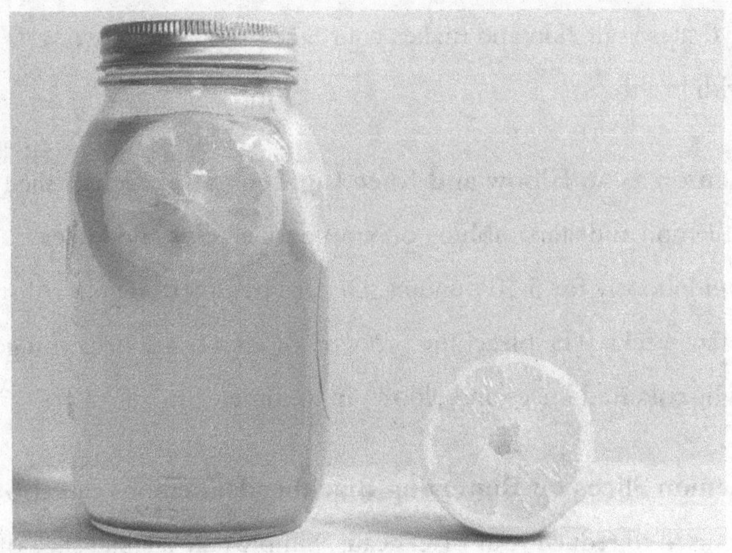

Lemon Juice for Treating Dandruff and Dry Scalp: Take two spoonfuls each of sea salt, olive oil and lemon juice. Mix all the ingredients well. Rub this mixture on your hair scalp for 8-10 minutes and then wash your hair with a mild shampoo. Do this once a week to get dandruff-free hair.

Lemon Juice for Premature Greying of Hair: Heat some coconut oil mildly and add lemon juice (squeezed from one lemon) to it. Mix well and apply the mixture evenly on your hair. Massage your scalp for 10 minutes. Wait for half an hour and then wash your hair with the help of a mild shampoo. This is an effective treatment to prevent premature greying.

Lemon Juice as a Face Moisturizer: Take few drops of coconut water with few drops of lemon juice and apply it on your face as a moisturizer. This is a natural moisturizer which hydrates your skin and makes your face bright and glowing with health. .

Lemon as an Elbow and Knee Lightener: Take a half slice of lemon and start rubbing on your dark elbows and knees continuously for 5-10 minutes. Do this treatment regularly for a few weeks. The bleaching property of lemon will help you get light-coloured knees and elbows in no time.

Lemon Slices for Removing Blackheads: Lemons can also be used to reduce your blackheads. Simply take a small slice of lemon and start rubbing it on your blackheads. After 10 minutes wash your face with water. Your face will immediately be cleared of blackheads.

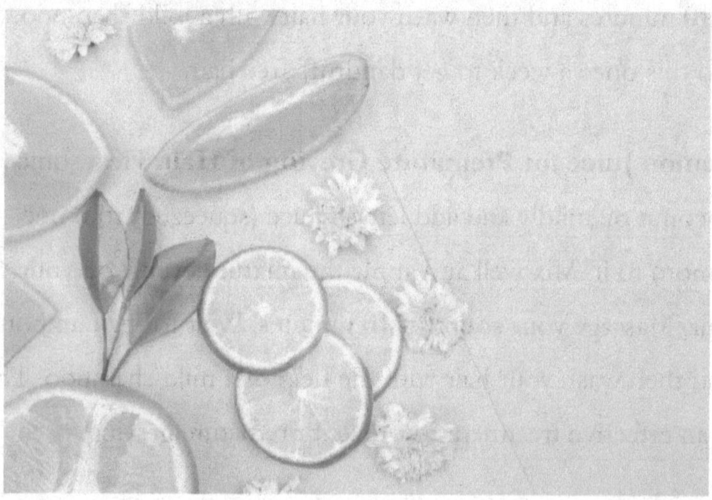

Lemon Juice as a Teeth Whitener: Mix baking soda with lemon juice and apply it on your teeth as toothpaste. Rub with toothbrush and rinse off. This treatment will provide you with healthy gums and white teeth.

Lemon Juice for Lips: You can make your own lip scrub by using lemon. Mix one spoonful of brown sugar in lemon juice taken from one large lemon. Use this scrub on your lips as a lip scrub regularly. This treatment will eventually remove all the dead cells from your lips and make them naturally pink and soft.

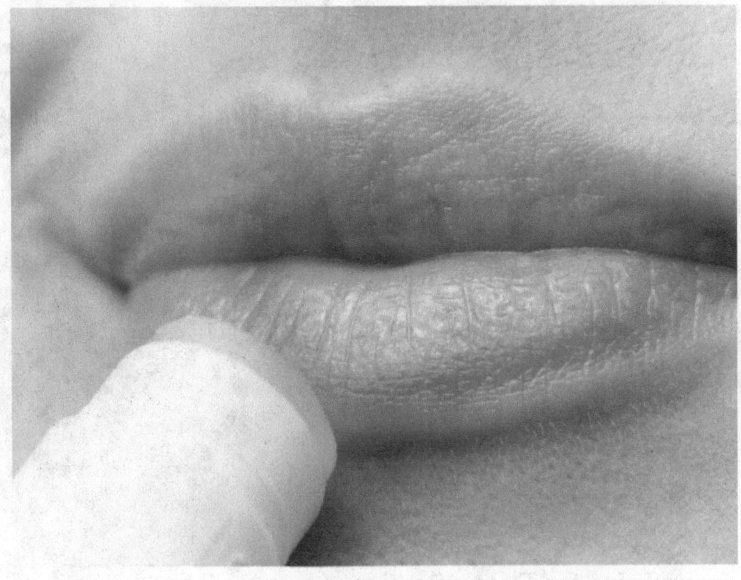

Lemon Juice for Healthy Nails: Take a bowl of warm water and add a few drops of olive oil in it. Now add lemon juice (squeezed from one large lemon) into the water. Mix the water before soaking the nails in it. Keep the nails soaked in water for 15-20 minutes. This treatment is the best way to fix dry and brittle nails.

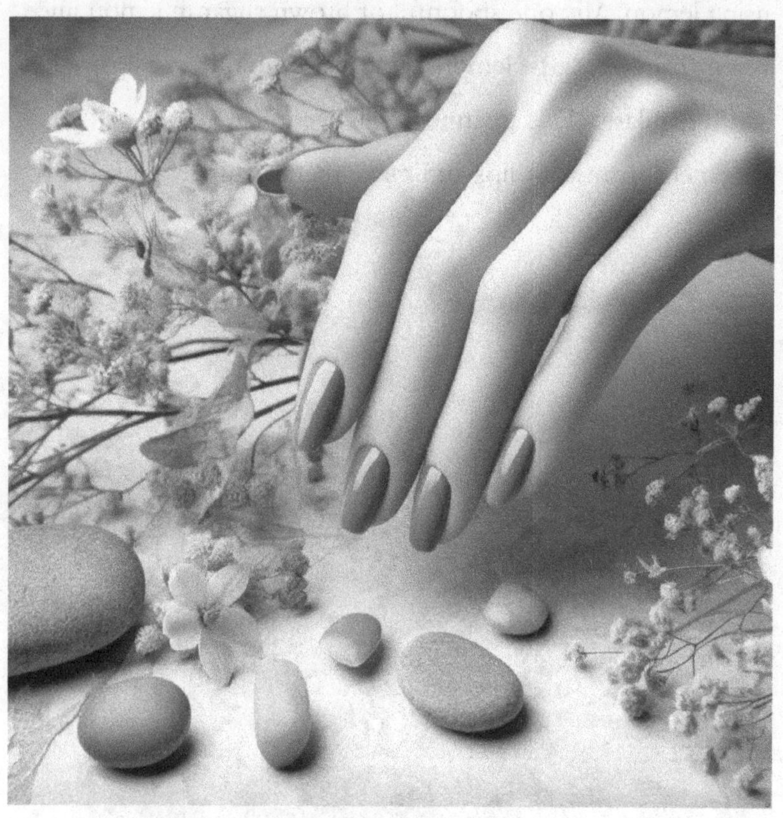

Lemon Juice for Detoxification: Lemon juice may be used as a part of your detox diet program.

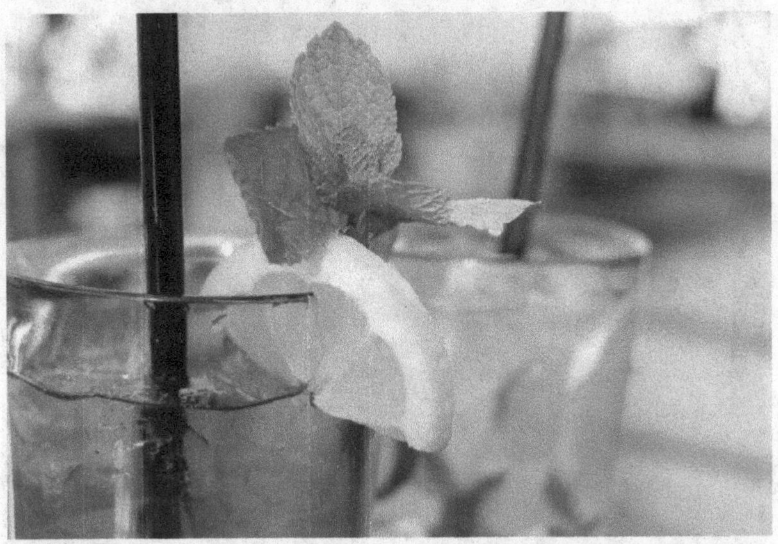

Lemon Juice as An Ingredient in Face Masks: If you make any kind of face masks (with any of the natural ingredients such as turmeric powder, bengal gram powder, honey, oatmeal etc.) lemon juice can be added as a bleaching agent.

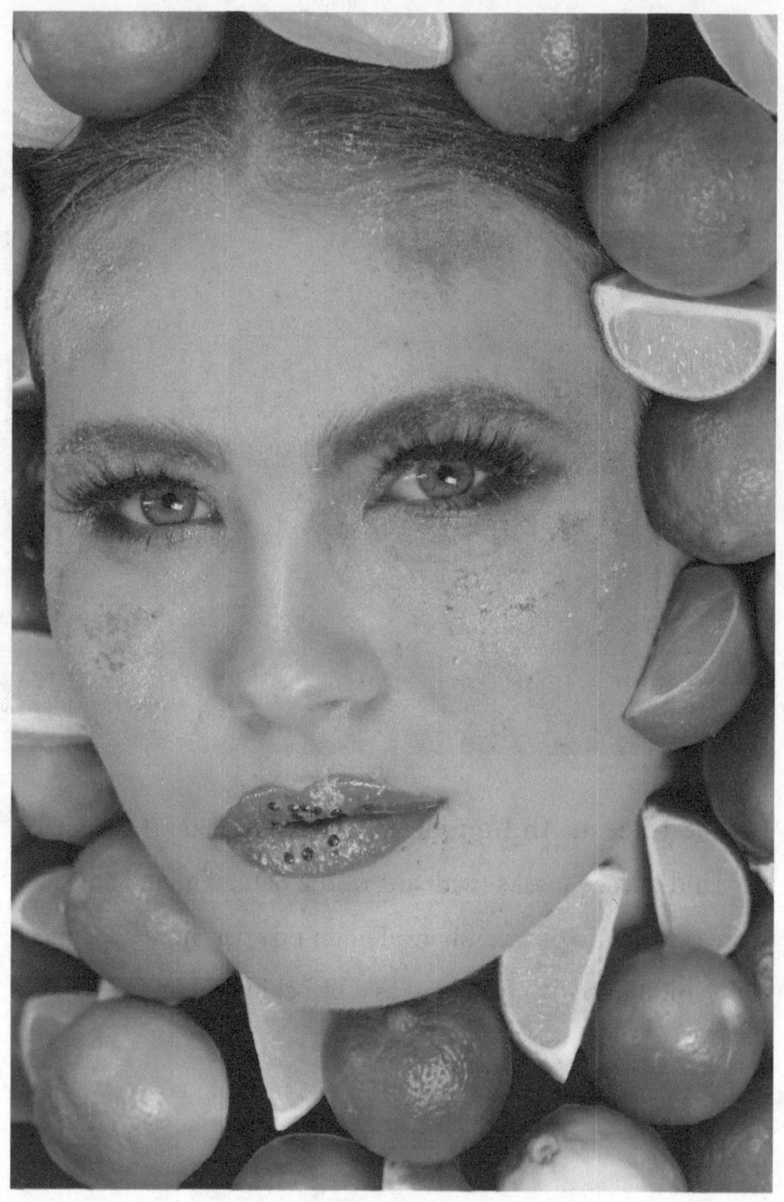

Oranges and Grapefruits As Natural Cosmetics

Orange is considered as a beauty food which is suitable for both as a food and a natural cosmetic for all age groups.

Orange Slices for Treating Facial Acne: Rubbing the face with orange slices regularly will help you diminish the occurrence of facial acne and pimples.

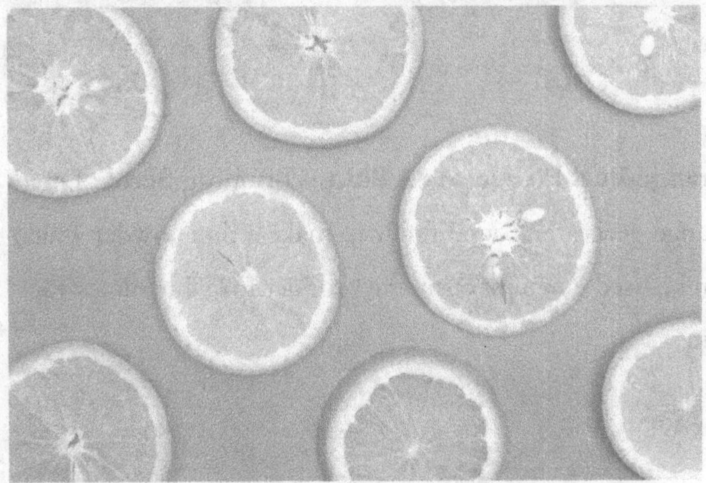

Orange Juice for Glowing Skin: Take two tablespoons of orange juice and one tablespoon each of honey and baking soda. Mix the ingredients well and after that, apply this mixture on skin. Leave it on for half an hour before washing it off with cold water. Regular use of this natural cosmetic will give you better results.

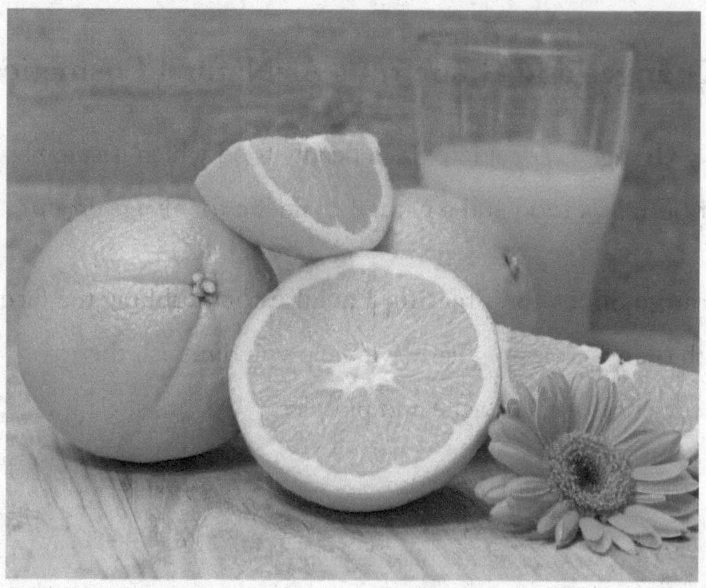

Orange Peel Powder As A Skin Whitening Scrub: Dried orange peels are ground finely to make a fine powder which can be used a natural cosmetic product for whitening your skin.

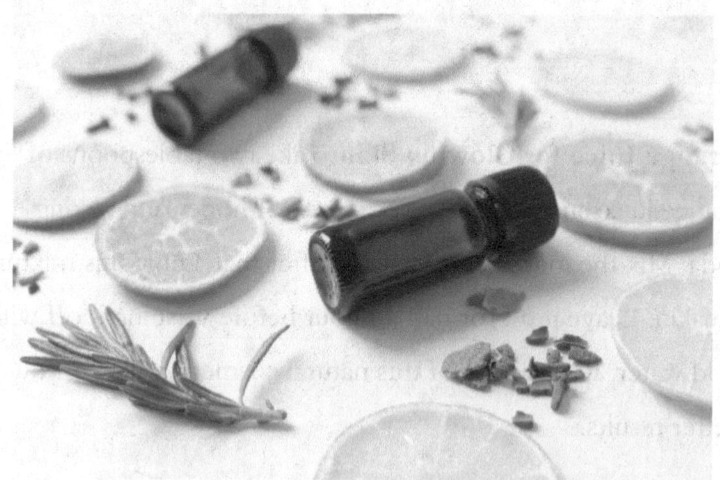

Orange Scrub for Cleansing Facial Skin: Whole parts of the orange fruits may be used to make an aromatic facial scrub.

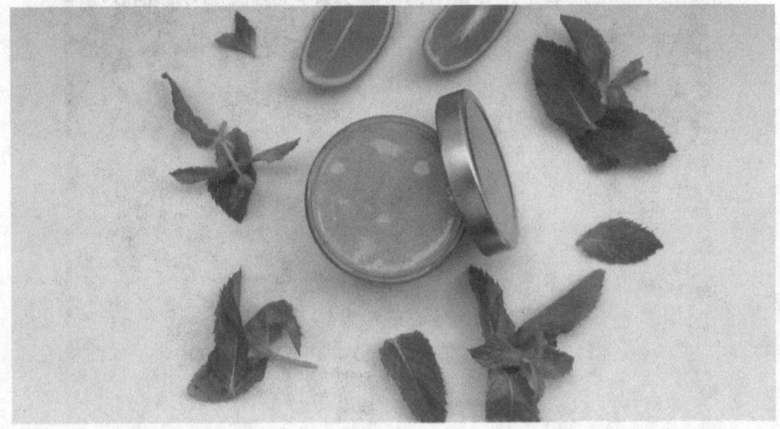

Papayas As Natural Cosmetics

Papaya is an incredibly healthy fruit. It is full of antioxidants that can help you reduce inflammation, fight diseases and help you look young. Papaya is a low-calorie fruit and is good for body weight management. Papaya fruit is used for many cosmetic purposes as well. Some papaya-based natural cosmetics and their preparation process are given below in detail. :

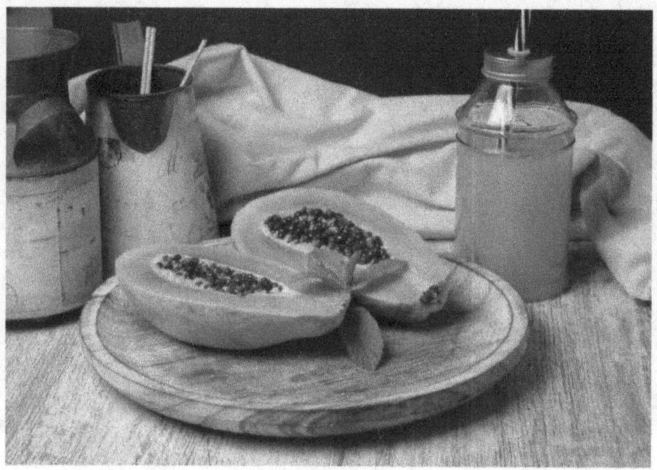

Papaya for Moisturizing Skin: For moisturizing your skin, mash one cup of chopped papaya fruit. Now add two tablespoons of honey to it. Mix the ingredients well and make a smooth paste by stirring continuously. Apply this paste evenly on your face and neck. Let it sit there for 20 minutes and then wash it off with cold water. This beauty treatment imparts instant glow to the face and neck.

Papaya for Treating Dark Circles around the Eyes: Papaya can help to get rid of dark circles of the eyes. Take half cup of mashed papaya fruit and half cup of grated cucumber. Mix them well. Apply this paste around the eyes on the dark circles and leave it for 10 minutes. After 10 minutes rub your eyes gently with your fingertips. Wipe the paste with a clean cloth and wash the eyes with lukewarm water. Repeat this beauty treatment daily until the dark circles are gone.

Papaya for Removing Skin Tanning: Take half cup of mashed papaya, ¼ cup of yogurt, one teaspoon of rose water and a pinch of turmeric powder. Mix them well. Now apply it on your tanned skin and leave it for 15 minutes. After that, wash your skin with cold water and dry with a towel. Regular use of this treatment will ultimately provide you with a tan-free glowing skin.

Papaya as a Hair Conditioner: For making papaya-based hair conditioner, you need ½ of a fully ripe papaya fruit. Mash the fruit thoroughly and then add ½ cup of coconut oil and one tablespoon of honey. Mix the ingredients well to make a paste. Apply this paste as a mask on your hair and leave it for 30-40 minutes. After that, rinse the hair off with water and shampoo. This beauty treatment helps to reduce the hair loss while promoting strong hair growth.

Papaya for Treating Dry Skin: Take ½ cup of mashed

papaya fruit, 2 teaspoons of milk and one tablespoon of honey. Mix them well and make a paste. Apply this paste as a mask on your face. Leave it for 15 minutes and then wash it off with cold water. Use this treatment twice a week for better results.

Papaya for Treating Acne: Take ½ cup of mashed papaya, 1 teaspoon of honey, 1 teaspoon of lemon juice and 1 teaspoon of sandalwood powder (optional). Mix all the ingredients properly. Apply this mask on your face and neck. Leave it for 10-15 minutes and rinse it off with cold water.

Papaya to Tighten Skin Pores: Take ½ cup of mashed papaya fruit and one egg white. Mix them well and make a paste. Apply this paste on your face. After 15 minutes, wash it off with cold water. Use this mask once a week. This treatment could help tone the skin and tighten the pores.

Papaya for Treating Oily Skin: Take one ripe papaya. Cut it into pieces and mash it with orange juice of 6-7 pieces of orange. Mix the ingredients well to make a smooth paste. Apply the paste on your face and wait for 15 minutes. After that wash your face with cold water. Do this twice a week. This mask will help to reduce the excess oil from your face.

Pomegranates As Natural Cosmetics

Pomegranate fruit is known for its rich iron and antioxidant contents. Drinking pomegranate juice regularly can help boosting your immunity and maintaining your dental health. It will also help you maintain the required iron content of your body. However, pomegranates aren't just for eating or drinking purposes. These fruits are excellent beauty aids and can also be used on our skin for making it healthier.

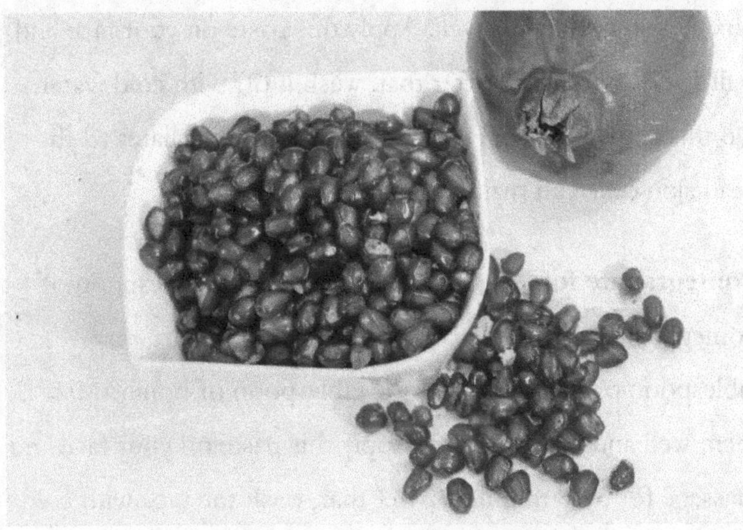

Pomegranate for Treating Sun Tan: Take a handful of pomegranate seeds and crush them properly to make a smooth powder. Mix this powder with half a spoonful of lemon juice to make a paste. Apply this paste as a mask on your face. After 30 minutes, wash off the mask with water. Do it twice or thrice in a week. This is an excellent skin-whitening beauty treatment.

Pomegranate for Moisturized Skin: Take one spoonful of powdered pomegranate seeds and one spoonful of honey. Mix the ingredients well to make a paste. Apply this paste on your face as a mask and then wait for 30 minutes before washing it off with cold water. Do this thrice a week for a perfectly moisturized facial skin.

Pomegranate for Glowing Skin: Take 2 tablespoons of pomegranate seed oil, 1 tablespoon of green papaya powder, 1 teaspoon of grape seed oil and 1 teaspoon grape seed extract. Mix all the ingredients well. Apply this paste on your face and wait for half an hour. After that, wash it off with cold water. Do this twice a week. This face pack gently exfoliates all the dead skin cells and makes your skin smooth.

Pomegranate for Treating Acne: Take one tablespoon of pomegranate seed paste, one tablespoon of yogurt, one tablespoon of green tea and one tablespoon of honey. Mix them well and make a paste. Apply this paste on your face and massage for 5-10 minutes. After that, wash the face with cold water. Do this twice a week. This mask will brighten up your face and prevent all possible acne-breakouts.

Pomegranate for Youthful Skin: Take 1 tablespoon of pomegranate seed powder and 1 tablespoon of cocoa powder. Mix it well to make a paste. Add water if the consistency is too thick. Apply the paste as a mask on your face. Wait until the mask is dry. Then wash it off with cold water. Do this twice a week for better results. This mask will keep the skin glowing and youthful.

Pomegranate for Flawless Skin: Take 3 tablespoons of yogurt and half a cup of pomegranate seeds. Make a smooth paste of pomegranate seeds. Add yogurt and blend them properly. Apply the paste on your face and wait for 20 minutes. Then wash it off. Apply this pack twice a week. This pack makes your skin soft and blemish-free.

Pomegranate for Revitalizing Your Skin: Take half a cup of pomegranate seeds and two tablespoons of oatmeal powder. Grind the pomegranate seeds to make a paste. Mix the oatmeal powder with pomegranate seed paste and blend the mixture well to make a smooth paste. Apply this paste as a mask on your face and massage with gentle circular strokes. Leave it for 30 minutes. Then rinse off with cold water. Do this once a week. This beauty treatment rejuvenates and revitalizes the facial skin.

Pomegranate for Wrinkles: Take half a cup of pomegranate seed paste, one tablespoon of rice flour and 3-4 drops of almond oil in a bowl and mix them well to make a paste. Apply this paste thoroughly all over the face and neck. Wait for 30 minutes and then wash with cold water. Do this twice a week. This face pack tones your face and neck and also reduces the signs of aging. This treatment also keeps the skin moisturized and hydrated.

Pomegranate Peel for Dry Skin: Dry pomegranate peel in the sun and grind it to make a smooth powder. Take two spoonfuls of pomegranate peel powder, one tablespoon of gram flour and two tablespoons of milk cream in a bowl. Mix them properly and make a smooth paste. Spread the paste evenly all over your face. After 20 minutes wash it off with water. Do this twice a week. This face mask is a good treatment for curing dry skin.

Pomegranate Peel for Dull Skin: Take three tablespoons of pomegranate peel powder, one tablespoon of lemon juice and two tablespoons of rose water in a bowl. Mix the ingredients well to make a paste. Apply the paste as a mask on your face and neck. Leave it for 20 minutes and then wash it off with cold water. Do this twice a week. This face pack brightens your skin tone. You will notice the difference right from the first usage.

Pomegranate Peel as a Facial Scrub: Pomegranate peel can help in removing dead skin, black and white heads from your face when it is used as a scrubber. For making this facial scrub, take two tablespoons of pomegranate peel powder and one spoon of brown sugar in a bowl. Add one spoon of honey, one spoon of avocado oil and mix all the ingredients well to make a scrub. Now apply this scrub on your face and massage thoroughly before washing it off with water. Do this regularly to get a smooth supple skin.

Pomegranate Peel for Treating Hair Loss and Dandruff: Pomegranate peels can also help you fight hair loss and prevent the growth of dandruff. Add one or two pinches of pomegranate peel powder in your hair oil before applying it on your hair. After oiling your hair, massage thoroughly from the hair roots. After 2 hours of oiling, wash your hair with a mild shampoo.

Pomegranate for Treating Sore Throat: Pomegranate peel powder can help you to soothe your sore throat. Take a handful of pomegranate peel powder and ass it in boiling water. Now strain the water and allow it to cool for a while. Then gargle with this water every few hours to get relief from sore throat and tonsil pains.

Walnuts As Natural Cosmetics

Walnuts are rich in omega-3 fats and antioxidants. Eating walnuts regularly may improve brain health also. Walnuts may be used as beauty foods as well. It is a well-established fact that regular consumption of walnuts may help hair and nails grow stronger and longer. Some of the home-made natural cosmetics prepared by using walnuts are illustrated in details as below:

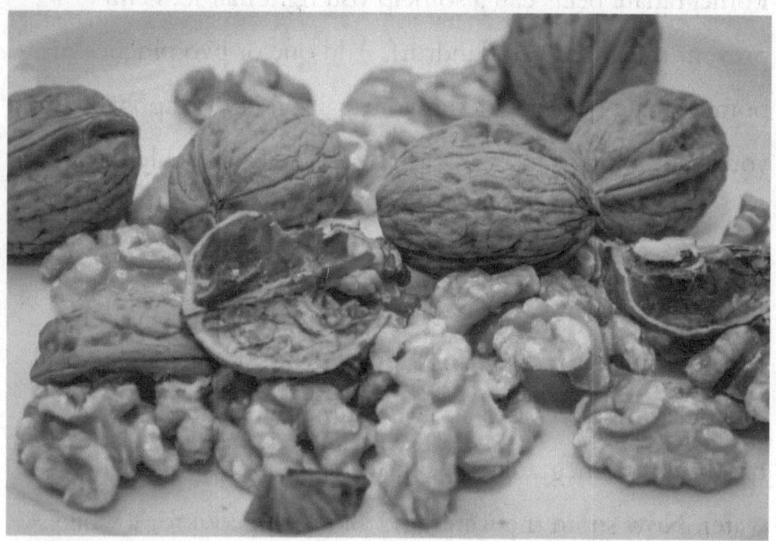

Walnut Face Scrub: Grind the shell of walnuts finely to make a smooth powder. Mix this powder with one tablespoon of coconut oil and few drops of rose water. Mix the ingredients well to make a paste and apply this paste as a scrub on your face and neck. Massage it gently for 5-10 minutes. Then rinse off with cold water. Do this testament once a week for few weeks for getting enhanced skin tone and glowing complexion.

Walnut for Skin Whitening: Take one tablespoon of walnut kernels powder, one tablespoon of mashed ripe papaya and one teaspoon of turmeric in a bowl. Mix them well and make a smooth paste. Apply the paste on your face and neck and wait for 15-20 minutes. Then wash it with cold water. Apply this mask twice a week for a few weeks for getting a younger and radiant looking skin.

Walnuts for Damaged Skin: Take one tablespoon of walnut powder and mix it with 2 tablespoons of yogurt. Make a smooth paste. Apply this paste on your face and let it dry completely before rinsing off with warm water.

Walnut for Removing Skin Tanning: Mix one teaspoonful of walnut powder with 2 teaspoonful of rose water. Now add one spoonful each of olive oil, lemon juice and honey. Make a smooth paste and apply it on your face. Leave it for 20 minutes and then wash it off with water. This will give you clear, fresh and toned uptight looking skin.

Walnut for Hair Loss: The best way to take the complete benefit of walnut for reducing hair loss is to eat a handful of walnuts daily. This will make your hair long, strong and healthy hair.

Walnut Oil for Healthy Scalp: For making your scalp healthy you just have to massage your scalp with walnut oil. Good massage will make your hair nourish from the roots.

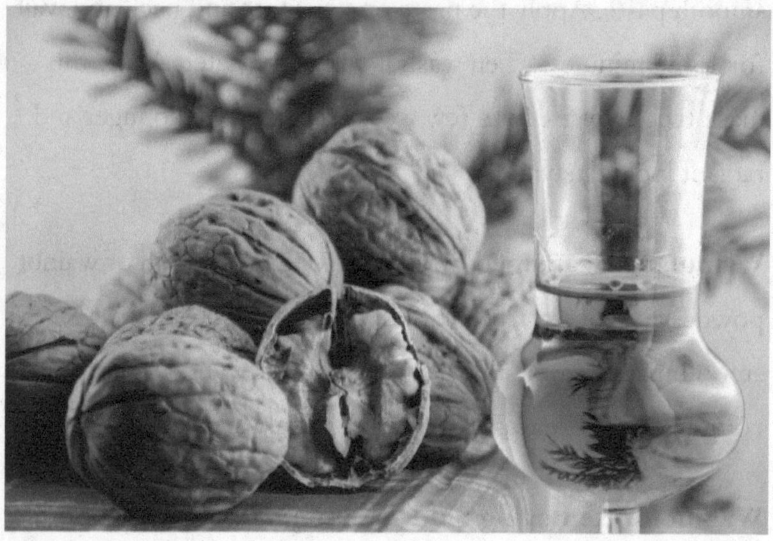

Walnuts as a Hair Dye: For using walnuts as a hair dye, first of all, crush about 10-15 walnut shells and keep them soaked in boiling water for half an hour. Cool the liquid and strain the shells. With the help of a cotton ball, apply the liquid over those strands of hair that you wish to dye. Leave it on for half an hour and rinse with cool water, followed by a mild shampoo and conditioner.

Beetroots As Cosmetics

Beetroots are one of the healthiest vegetables. Beetroot juice acts as a blood purifier, which keeps your skin glowing and healthy. Beetroot helps in clearing blemishes and evens out your skin tone while giving it a natural glow. It also strengthens hair follicles and prevents hair loss. Consuming beetroot or beetroot juice helps to improve the health of your hair. An account of some natural cosmetics that can be prepared by using beetroots is given below

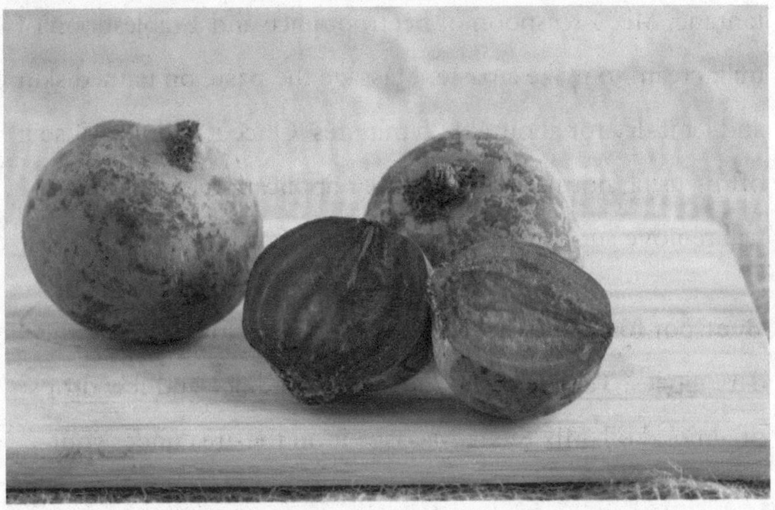

Beetroot Juice for Dry Skin: Take 1 teaspoon of raw milk, 2-3 drops of coconut oil and 2 teaspoons of beetroot juice. Mix the ingredients properly to make a smooth liquid. Gently massage it on your face. Let it stay for 10 minutes. Later wash it off with plain water and see the results.

Beetroot for Skin Brightening: Take 2 teaspoons of orange peel powder and 1 teaspoon of beetroot juice. Mix the ingredients together to make a thick paste. Apply it evenly on your face. Then wash it off with cold water. Apply this on alternate days for better results.

Beetroot for Tanning: Beetroot can help you get rid of tanning. Mix 1 teaspoon of beetroot juice and 1 tablespoon of milk cream to make a paste. Massage the paste on tanned skin and let it dry for about 20-25 minutes. Once it is done, rinse it off by using normal water. Regular application of this cream will remove sun-tan from skin within a few days.

Beetroot for Dark Circles: Beetroot helps in lightening the dark circles. Take 1 teaspoon of beetroot juice and few drops of almond oil. Mix them. Massage it on the area under your eyes. Let it sit for 15 minutes. Then wash it off with cold water. Repeat the beauty treatment for a week or more. Dark circles will disappear within a week.

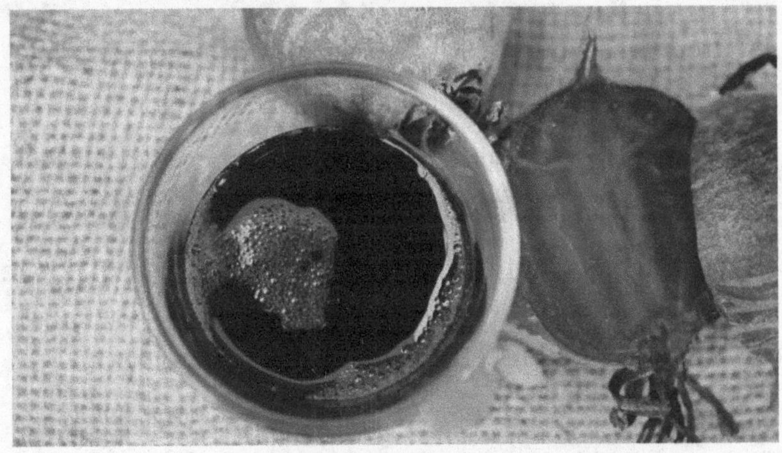

Beetroot for Smooth Skin: Take 3 tablespoons of yogurt and 4 teaspoons of beetroot juice. Mix the ingredients well to make a paste. Apply this paste on your face and neck evenly. Leave it there for 8-10 minutes. After that gently massage the face and neck before rinsing it off with warm water.

Beetroot for Enhancing Complexion: Grate a beetroot slice and mash it thoroughly to make a paste. Now apply this paste on your face and neck. Leave it for 10-15 minutes before washing off. Use this mask regularly to get a natural pinkish glow to the complexion.

Beetroot for Beautiful Lips: If your lips are flaky, chapped or losing the moisture, then beetroot juice is the best solution. Just apply some amount of beetroot juice onto your lips and let it sit there for a few minutes before washing it off. You can also mix sugar with grated beetroot to exfoliate dead cells from your lips.

Beetroot for Dandruff: Take equal parts of vinegar or neem water and beetroot juice and mix the liquid well. Now apply this solution on your hair. After one or two hours, wash it off with a mild shampoo. This beauty treatment is very effective in treating itchy dandruff.

Beetroot for Wrinkles: Take a little bit of beetroot juice, honey and milk. Mix them well. Apply this solution on your face evenly and le t it dry before washing it off. Do this beauty treatment once or twice a week for a few weeks to get a wrinkle-free facial skin.

Beetroot for Acne and Pimples: Mix equal parts of beetroot juice and tomato juice. Now apply it evenly on your face. Leave it dry for at least 15 minutes. Wash it off with cold water. Do this beauty treatment repeatedly until your face is free of acnes and pimples.

Beetroot as Red Hair Dye: Mix half cup of carrot juice and half cup of beetroot juice to make a red-colour natural hair dye. Use the solution to massage the hair from the hair roots. Use this dye liberally on the hair to get the desired red colour. After applying the dye, wait for one or two hours to dry it completely. After that wash the hair with a mild shampoo. This hair treatment will leave your hair with a natural reddish or brownish colour.

Carrots As Cosmetics

Carrots are rich in vitamins, minerals and dietary fiber. Carrots help to maintain healthy cholesterol. It also helps to prevent heart-related diseases and in promoting eye health. Carrots are also known for their beauty benefits as well. A list of some carrot-based natural cosmetic preparations is given below:

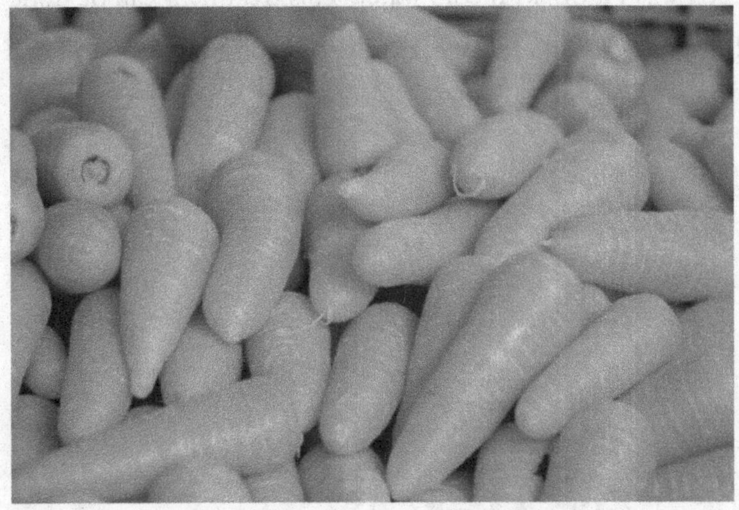

Carrot Face Mask for Skin Brightness: Boil some carrots and let it cool. Now blend the boiled carrots into a smooth paste. Take a ripe papaya fruit and scoop the flesh out to make a thin paste. Mix papaya paste and carrot paste well by adding some milk and mix it well until a fine cream is made. Now apply this cream on your face and neck evenly. Wait for 20-30 minutes. After that, wash your face mildly with lukewarm water and then dab a towel on your face to dry.

Do this beauty treatment regularly to flaunt a naturally-bright facial skin always.

Carrot Face Mask for Dull and Dry Skin: Grate 2-3 carrots thinly and strain the juice out of the grated carrots. Now mix one tablespoon each of honey and milk cream with the carrot juice to make a cream. Apply this cream evenly on your face and neck by using a soft brush. Leave it for 15-20 minutes. Then wash it off with cold water. This treatment can be done thrice a week for a few weeks to get the best results.

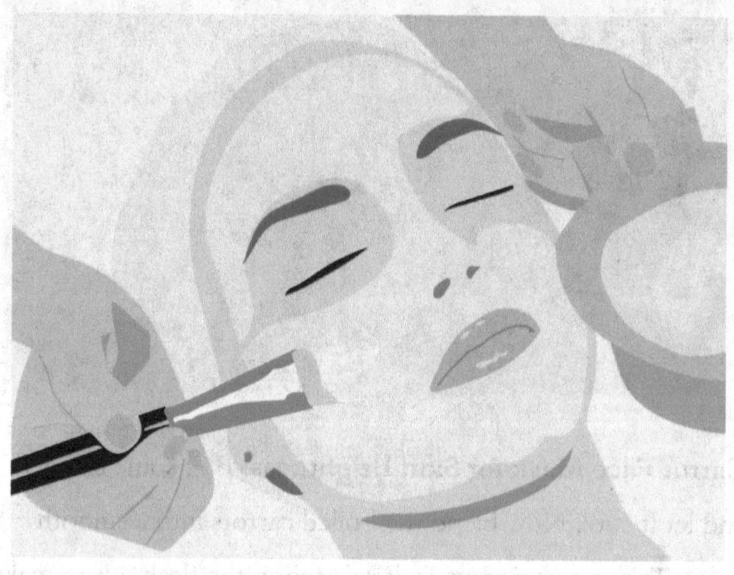

Carrots for Removing Acne and Pimples: Grate two carrots thinly and then strain the juice out of it. Mix three teaspoons of carrot juice with a teaspoon of honey and 2-3 pinches of cinnamon powder. Use this mixture as a face pack on a dry facial skin to get the best results. After applying the face pack wait for 20 minutes and then wash it off with cold water. Do not use soap or face wash immediately to avoid any kind of irritability on the skin.

Carrots for Oily Skin: Take one small cup of carrot juice and mix it with one tablespoon each of curd, gram flour, and lemon juice. Mix the ingredients well to make a thick paste. Apply this paste as a mask evenly on your face and neck and wait for half an hour. Then wash it off with lukewarm water. Excess oil from the facial skin can be removed by this beauty treatment.

Carrot Face Pack for Clear Glowing Complexion: Mix equal parts of carrot juice, yogurt and egg white. Mix all the ingredients well to make a smooth cream. Apply this cream on face and neck evenly with finger tips and wait for 15 minutes to let the face pack dry. After that, wash the pack off with lukewarm water. Carrot face pack helps to remove dirt and dead skin cells from the face thus giving way to a fresh-looking facial skin with clear and glowing complexion.

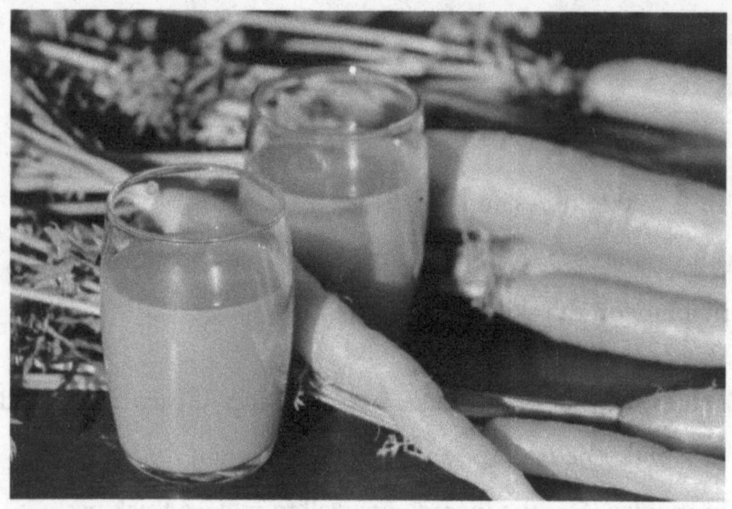

Carrot-Based Sun Protection Spray: Carrots helps to protect our skin against UV rays and also helpful in removing sun tan. Take equal parts of carrot juice and rose water and mix them well. Now fill the mixture in a spray bottle. Spray it on your face and body daily. It will keep the skin hydrated and also protect the skin from the harmful rays of the sun.

Carrot-Based Body Cram for Anti-Ageing: Take equal parts of carrot juice and aloe vera gel in a bowl. Mix the ingredients well to make a smooth cream. Apply this cream on face and body on regular basis in order to fight the signs of early ageing.

Carrots for Nourishing Your Hair: Grate a carrot finely. Take a small glass jar and put the grated carrot in it. Now fill the jar with olive oil before closing its lid. Store this jar in a dark corner of the house for a week. When the oil has turned into orange colour, strain the oil and transfer it into a clean container. Use this hair oil to massage your scalp and hair regularly. After massaging the hair from the roots, wait for at least half an hour before washing it off with a mild shampoo. Use this hair oil regularly for a few months for getting stronger, longer and healthier hair.

Carrot for Repairing Split Hair and for Promoting Hair Growth: Chop one carrot and one banana into small pieces. Blend them in a food processor along with two tablespoons of yogurt. Take out the perfectly blended ingredients and use it as a hair mask. Apply this mask all over your hair thoroughly and evenly. After applying it, cover your hair with a shower cap and leave it on for 30 minutes. After that, wash it off with a mild shampoo. Follow this routine once a week for a few weeks to get better results.

Carrot-Based Hair Mask for Soft and Shiny Hair: This mask will hydrate your scalp and moisturize your hair to make it softer and fuller. Carrot also helps to boost hair growth and promote hair health. Take a small cup of carrot paste (grind the grated carrots finely to make it a paste) Mix it with two tablespoons of coconut oil to make a paste. Apply this paste as a mask all over your scalp and hair thoroughly and evenly. Leave the hair mask on for 20-30 minutes. Finally, wash it off with a mild shampoo. Follow this routine once a week for a few weeks in order to get the best results.

Carrot Hair Spray: A carrot hair spray could be a convenient way of boosting your hair health. This spray also helps to prevent hair loss. Blend two carrots in a blender and strain the paste to extract the juice. Fill half the spray bottle with the carrot juice and remaining part with aloe vera juice. Shake well. Spray this solution all over your scalp and then massage the head with your finger tips for 10 minutes. After that, wait for 30 minutes or more before washing it off with a mild shampoo. Follow this routine twice a week for a few months for promoting your hair growth and scalp health.

Cucumbers As Natural Cosmetics

Cucumbers are moisture-rich vegetables and consuming them regularly will keep the skin hydrated and healthy always. Cucumbers can be used as external beauty aids as well because of their cooling and soothing properties. Applying these vegetables on our skin can help to reduce sunburn pain, swelling and damaged skin. A list of various cucumber-based natural cosmetics is given below:

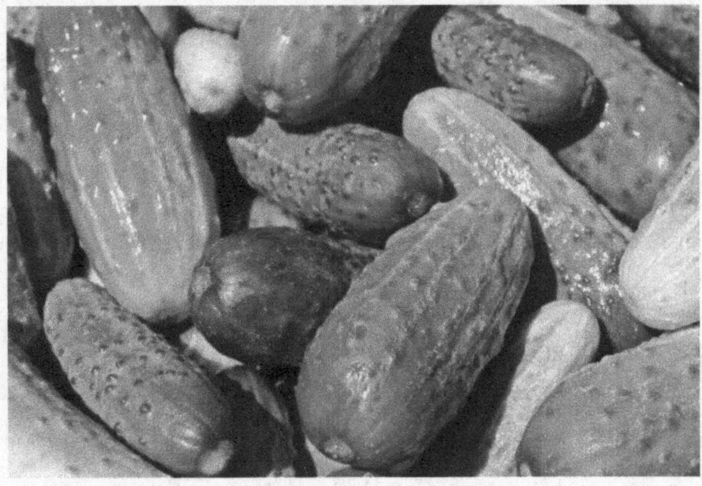

Cucumber for Removing Skin Tan: Cucumber juice helps to soothe the sun-tanned skin. Take a bowl and mix one tablespoon each of cucumber juice, lemon juice and rose water. Use this solution evenly all over the skin. Wait for 10 minutes. Then wash it off with cold water.

Cucumber for Repairing Dull Skin: Mix one tablespoon of cucumber juice with a teaspoon of lemon juice. Apply this cooling blend on your face daily. Let it sit for 10 minutes. Now use a wet towel to pat dry your skin. Cucumber gives new life to dull and lifeless skin and rejuvenates it due to its hydrating properties.

Cucumber Treats Blemishes: If you want to keep your blemishes and freckles away then wash your face daily with cucumber water. Another way to treat skin blemishes is the use of a cucumber-based cream.

Mix one tablespoon of oats with one small cup of cucumber pulp. Blend the ingredients well to make a cream. Apply the cream as a mask on your face. Wait for 20 -30 minutes. Then wash your face with cold water. This mask will exfoliate and keep your skin clear of blemishes and scars.

Cucumber for Dark Circles and Puffy Eyes: You can put thin cucumber slices on your dark circles and let it rest for eight to ten minutes. Rinse it off with cold water. If you want you can place two slices of cucumber directly on your eyes. This is a great way to refresh puffy and tired eyes. The best time to use cucumber slices on eyes is always after a good facial.

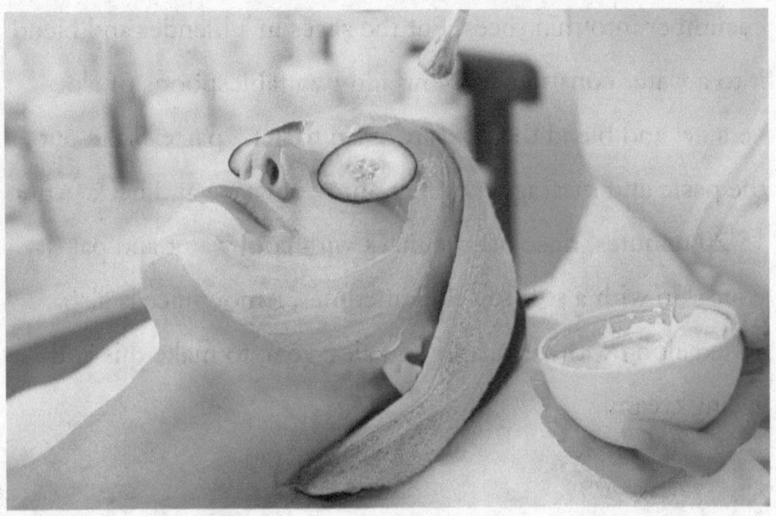

Cucumber for Irritated and Acne-Prone Skin: Blend ½ a cucumber and transfer it into a bowl. Now add one tablespoon of yogurt. Mix the ingredients well until a fine cream is made. Now spread an even layer of cream onto your skin. Let the mask dry for 15 - 20 minutes. Finally, wash the mask off with lukewarm water. This beauty treatment is the best natural remedy for irritated facial skin.

Cucumber for Removing Wrinkles: Take ¼ of a cucumber and blend it in a hand blender until it's slightly chunky. Apply the cucumber mash directly on to the facial skin and neck as a mask. Let the mask sit for 15-20 minutes before washing it off with lukewarm water. This beauty treatment is one of the best natural remedies for wrinkle-free facial skin.

Cucumber for Youthful Skin: Cucumber helps to soothe, hydrate and heal dry and old skin. Cut ½ of an unpeeled cucumber into thin slices. Put the slices in a blender and blend it to a water consistency. Now add two tablespoons of aloe vera gel and blend the mixture again to get a paste. Take out the paste and massage it evenly onto your face and neck. After 15-20 minutes, rinse off the mask with cool water and pat dry your skin with a soft towel. Sometimes, lemon juice is also added along with cucumber and aloe vera, to make this anti-ageing cream.

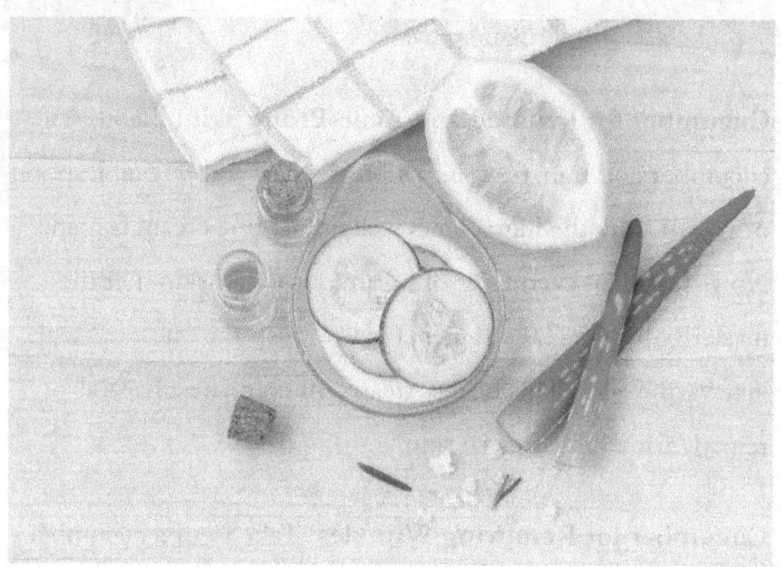

Cucumber Skin Lotion: Cucumber lotion helps to soothe and tighten the skin. It also helps to close open pores so dirt doesn't penetrate the skin. To make a cucumber lotion, all you have to do is blend together ½ a cucumber, 3 tablespoons of witch hazel and 2 tablespoons of mineral water. Blend all the ingredients well until the mixture is smooth and lotion-like. Take the lotion out and pour it through a strainer into a clean container. Close the container and store it in a dark corner of the house. Since shelf-life of all these natural cosmetics is very less, use them within a week. You can use this cucumber-based body lotion on daily basis.

Cucumber Hair Mask: To make a cucumber-based hair mask, all you have to do is take one egg, one tablespoon olive oil and half of a peeled cucumber. Put all the ingredients together in a food processor and blend them until you get a smooth paste. Use this paste as a hair mask. The mask should be applied evenly throughout the hair and leave it on for about 10-20 minutes. Then rinse the hair thoroughly with cold water. Repeated use of this hair mask will result in health and shiny hair.

Cucumber Facial: For doing a cucumber facial, you need a few long and fresh cucumbers. Slice them longitudinally into very thin slices so that they stick to the skin tightly. After massaging the face with a massage cream, place the cucumber slices one by one on the face and neck in such a manner that every inch of the skin should be covered with the slices. Let the slices sit on the face until they become dry. Finally, remove the cucumber slices and wash the face with lukewarm water. Cucumber facial is one of the best and natural anti-ageing facials that are available today.

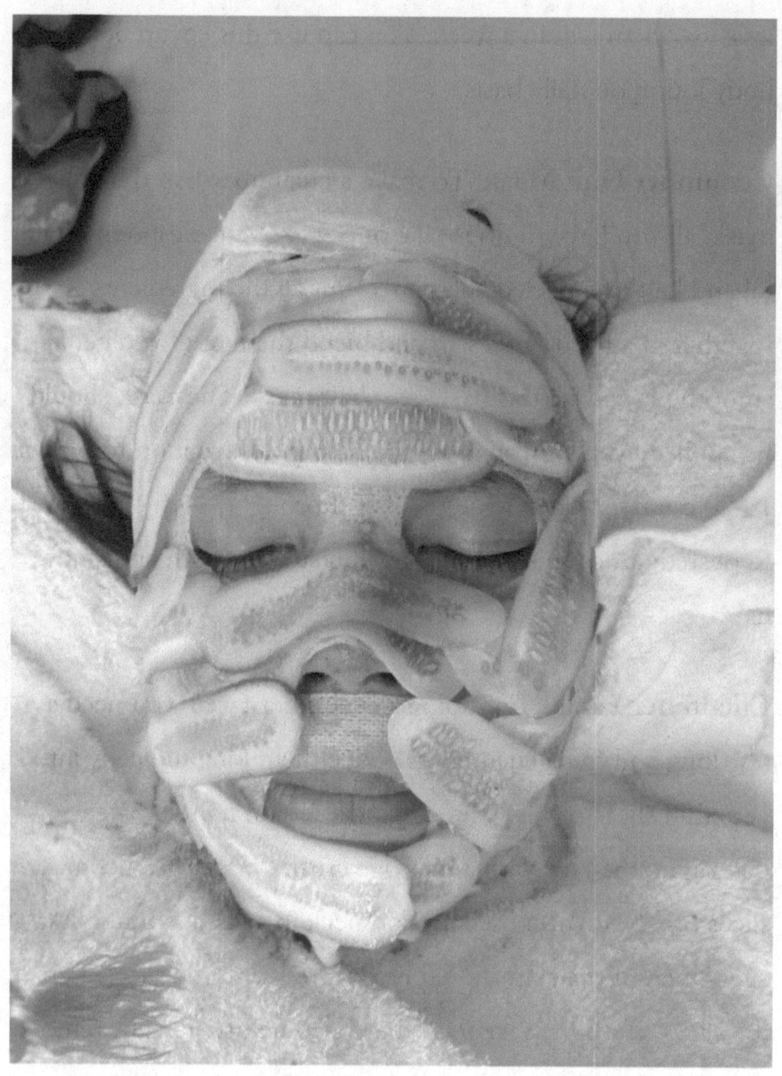

Onions as Natural Cosmetics

Onion is a common and popular bulb vegetable that can be found in every kitchen, anywhere in the world. Onions may also be used to treat ailments like headaches, heart diseases and mouth sores. Apart from these culinary and medicinal benefits of onions, some cosmetic benefits can also be derived from these super vegetables. A list of various natural-cosmetics that can be prepared from onions is given below:

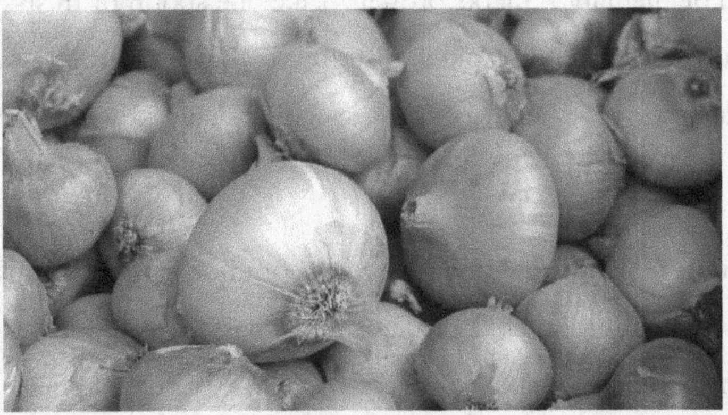

Onion Fight Hair Loss: Boil some water with an onion in it. Let it cool and then strain the liquid out of it. Use this liquid to rinse your hair before shampooing it to fight hair loss. This hair treatment will prevent the occurrence of dandruff on scalp and will also promote new hair growth.

Onion for Treating Sunburn: For treating your sunburn or any other minor burns, simply rub a sliced onion on it for a few minutes. It will also help in skin regeneration and in reducing burning and redness of skin.

Onion for Removing Skin Spots, Patches and Pigmentation: Onion helps to treat dark spots, ugly patches, and pigmentation marks on skin. Take one spoon of fresh onion juice and add a pinch of turmeric powder to it. Massage your face and other affected areas with it daily for a few days for better results.

Onion for Curing Acne: Acne is a common skin problem among many women. You can simply massage your face with some fresh onion juice or you can even add one tablespoon of olive oil/almond oil to it. Blend the ingredients well and apply on your skin. Do a mild massage for some time. After 15 minutes wash it off with cold water.

Tomatoes As Natural Cosmetics

Tomatoes are full of antioxidants which have been linked to many health benefits, including reduced risk of heart diseases and cancer. It is also helpful for skin and eye care. As a beauty food, tomato helps to cure large pores, acne, sunburn and dull skin. Some of the cosmetic uses of tomatoes are stated below:

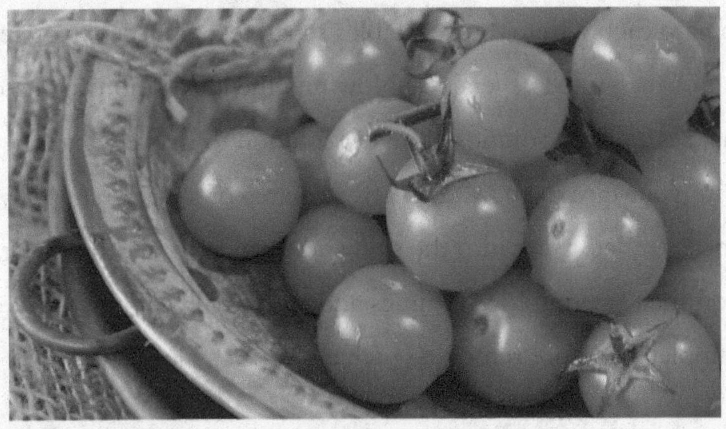

Tomato for Removing Blackheads: Take two teaspoons of rice flour and ¼ teaspoon of turmeric powder. Now add tomato juice to make a paste. Massage this paste gently on your face especially the blackhead-affected areas for a few minutes. Let the face pack dry. Once the face pack has dried enough, wash it off with lukewarm water.

Tomato for Skin Glow: Mix equal parts of tomato juice and honey. Apply this mixture on your face by using a cotton pad. Let it dry for 10-15 minutes. Then wash it off. This treatment is perfect to achieve that enviable healthy glow instantly.

Tomato for Acne-Free, Oil Free Skin: Mash a ripe tomato and mix it with some cucumber juice to make a thick paste. Now apply it directly on your skin by spreading it evenly to cover every inch of the skin surface. Let it dry and then wipe it away with a cotton ball.

Tomato for Removing Suntan: Take one potato and one tomato each. Grate the vegetables separately. Squeeze the juice out of the grated vegetables. Now mix the juices thoroughly to make a uniform solution. Use the solution to massage lightly onto your face or the suntan affected area of skin. First apply one layer, let it sink into the skin and then apply another layer. Continue layering for 4-5 times and then finally let it get dry completely before removing with a wet wash cloth.

Tomato as a Scrubber: You can prepare an effective scrubber by using tomato and red lentil. Soak a handful of lentil in water overnight. In the morning blend the red lentils with half of a fresh, red tomato. Blend until they make a smooth paste. Now use this paste as a scrub on the skin and leave it on for 5-6 minutes. Then wash it off with plenty of water. This beauty treatment is considered as one of the best home remedies for skin rejuvenation.

Tomato to Heal Skin Burns: Frozen tomato juice is very effective for healing and treating the skin burns. Just simply apply some frozen tomato juice on the affected areas. Leave it on for some time and then wash it off with cold water.

Tomato for Treating Sunburn: Take one fresh tomato and ½ cup of the curd in a blender. Blend the ingredients in the blender to make a paste. Take the perfectly blended paste out of the blender to use as a mask on the sunburns or other affected areas. After applying the mask, wait for 10-15 minutes and then wash it off with the cool water.

Tomato for Dark Circles: For treating your dark circles, dip a cotton ball in tomato juice and put it on dark circles of eyes. Wait for 10 minutes and then rinse it off with water. This is one of the best home remedies to lighten your dark circles.

Tomato as a Cure for Itchy Scalp and Dandruff: Take three small tomatoes and make a pulp of them. Now add two tablespoons of lemon juice into the pulp. Mix the ingredients well and make a smooth paste. Gently rub the paste on your scalp by using your finger tips. Leave it on for 30 minutes before you wash it off with cold water. Repeat this treatment twice a week for the better results.

Tomato for Thick Hair: In a bowl, blend on pulp from one ripe tomato and two tablespoons of castor oil until it forms a smooth paste. Warm this mixture slightly. Apply the mixture on your scalp evenly by using the finger tips and then start massaging the scalp for some time. After that, leave this hair mask on for 1-2 hours before washing it off by using a mild shampoo and conditioner. Repeat this treatment twice a week for the desired results.

Tomato for Hair Conditioning: In a bowl, take two ripe tomatoes and mash them completely. Add two tablespoons of honey to the mashed tomatoes and blend it until it forms a consistent paste. Leave the mixture as it is for a few minutes before you start applying it on your hair. After the application, cover your head with a shower cap. Wait for 30 minutes and then wash it off with cold water. Repeat this process once a week for the desired results.

Tomato for Treating Premature Grey Hair: To get rid of premature grey hair, just apply tomato pulp on your scalp and hair evenly and thoroughly. Leave it on for 20 minutes. Then wash it off with water and a shampoo.

Potatoes as Natural Cosmetics

Potatoes are used as vegetables and as a staple food in almost all countries across the globe. Though we all know various food preparations based on potatoes, most of us are quite ignorant about their beauty benefits when used as a natural cosmetic. So a list of some of the most popular potato-based natural cosmetics is given below for your understanding.

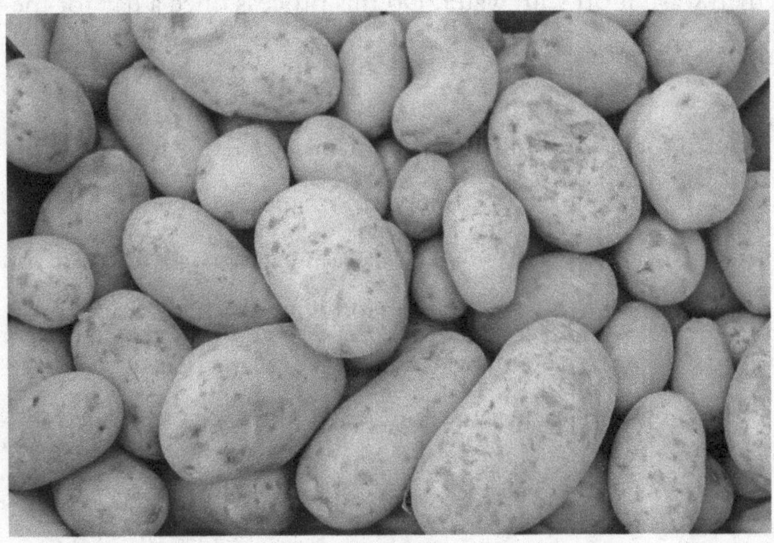

Potato for Skin Whitening: Mix three tablespoons of potato juice with two tablespoons of honey. Mix them well and apply it on your face and neck. Leave it for 10-15 minutes and then wash it off. Do this treatment daily for getting the best results.

Potato for Glowing Skin: Add two tablespoons of potato juice with two tablespoons of lemon juice. If you want you can add half a spoon of honey too. Mix them well and apply it on your face and neck. Lave it for 15 minutes and wash it off with water. Do this treatment every alternate day for the better results.

Potato for Removing Acne: Take one spoonful each of potato juice or pulp, tomato juice or pulp and honey. Mix them until you obtain a smooth paste. Apply it evenly on your face, focusing on the acne-affected area. Wait for 20 minutes and then wash it off with water. Do this process once a day for the better results.

Potato for Removing Pigmentation: Take one teaspoonful each of potato juice, rice flour, lemon juice and honey. Mix all the ingredients well to make a smooth paste. Apply it evenly on your face and neck. Leave it for some time to dry. Now scrub the dry face pack gently with the help of water. Clean your face thoroughly in a circular motion. Apply this face pack twice a week for the best results.

Potato for Removing Excess Oil from Skin: Take three boiled mashed potatoes, two tablespoons of milk, one tablespoon of oatmeal and one teaspoon of lemon juice. Mix all the ingredients well until you get a smooth paste. Apply this paste evenly on your face and neck. Leave it on for about 30 minutes. Then wash it off with lukewarm water. Do this treatment twice a week for a few weeks to get the best results.

Blackpepper as Natural Cosmetics

Black pepper helps to reduce acne due to its anti-inflammatory and antibacterial properties. When we apply pepper on our skin *with other ingredients* then it helps to loosen up the pores and facilitate the removal of blackheads and acne. (*Remember, never apply pepper directly on the skin; pepper is always used with other ingredients for cosmetic purposes*)

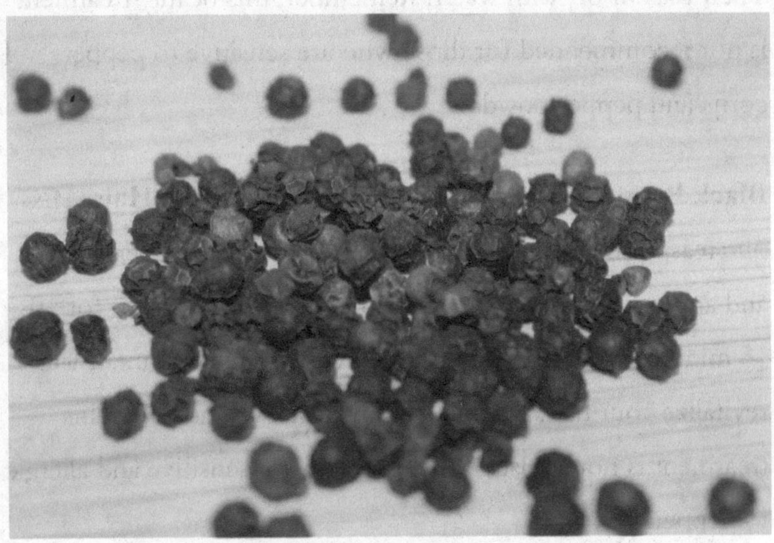

Black Pepper for Oral Health: Mix equal amounts of salt and pepper powder in water to make a paste. Rub the paste on your teeth for reducing toothache and increasing oral health.

Black Pepper Exfoliates the Skin: Black pepper can also be used as a scrub to remove dead skin cells and exfoliate the skin. Just take ½ teaspoon of powdered black pepper and one teaspoon of yogurt. Apply to your face. Wait for 20 minutes.

Then wash it off with water. Remember, this beauty treatment is not recommended for those who are sensitive to pepper corns and pepper powder.

Black Pepper Treats Dandruff and Revitalizes Hair: Mix one teaspoon each of lemon, honey, and black pepper powder and apply to your scalp and hair. Leave the mixture on for 10-15 minutes and rinse off with cold water. This treatment will revitalize your hair, making it shiny, lustrous and soft. This treatment is not advised for those who are sensitive and allergic to pepper.

Cinnamon as Natural Cosmetics

Cinnamon, when used externally creates a stimulus so strong that it draws blood to the surface of the skin, speeding up blood circulation and helps your skin breathe and hydrate and consequently eliminates acne and other skin problems.

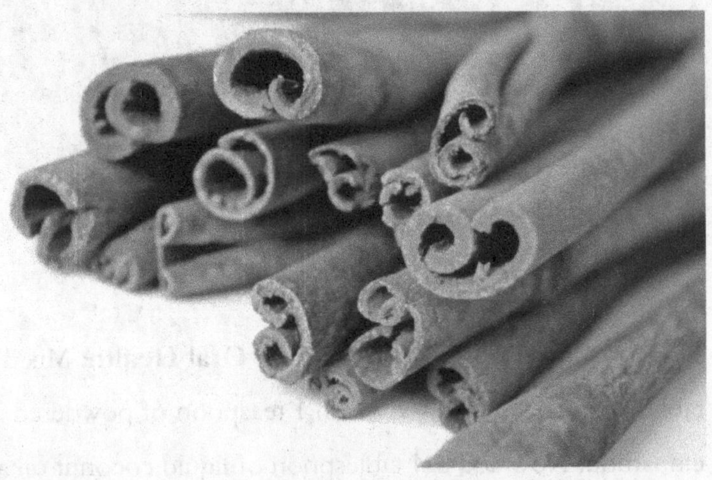

Cinnamon for Acne: Combine honey and cinnamon powder and create a thick paste. Apply it to pimples or problematic areas of skin. Leave the paste there for 15 minutes and then wash it off with cool or lukewarm water.

Cinnamon to Treat Bad Breath: Mix little honey and cinnamon powder with warm water. Use this mixture to gargle in the morning and night to treat bad breath.

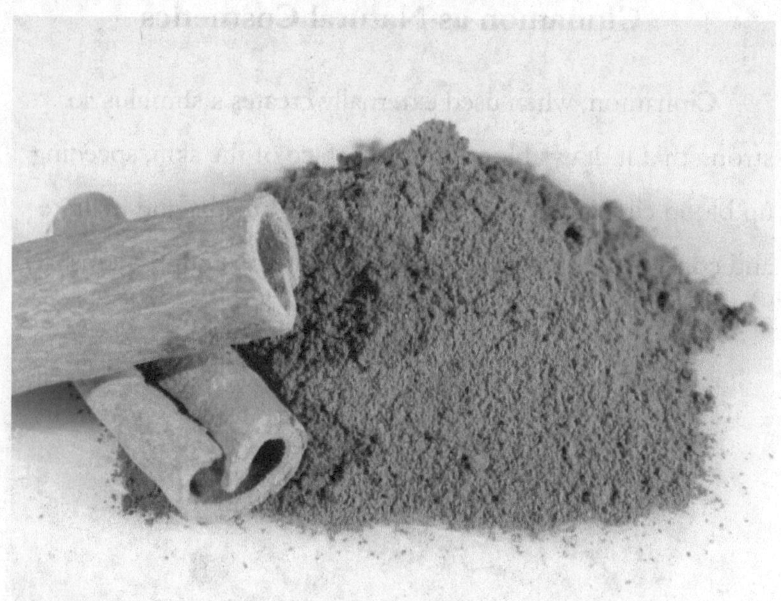

Natural Cinnamon Toothpaste for Oral Health: Mix 3 tablespoons of baking soda with 1 teaspoon of powdered cinnamon. Now add 3-4 tablespoon of liquid coconut oil and a few drops of peppermint essential oil to make a thick paste. Your cinnamon toothpaste is ready to use. Store this in a glass container in the fridge.

Cinnamon for Moisturizing Lips and Treating Dry Skin: Make a scrub by combining salt, olive oil, almond oil, honey and ground cinnamon. Apply this mixture on your lips and skin regularly to get the better results.

Cloves as Natural Cosmetics

Cloves are a powerful anti-aging ingredient used in most cosmetics. Clove oil helps in reducing the dullness of the skin. It also helps to prevent the appearance of fine lines and wrinkles. It removes the dead skin cells and helps in blood circulation, which indirectly or directly ensures a youthful and radiant looking skin. Let's see below how to use cloves to enhance our beauty.

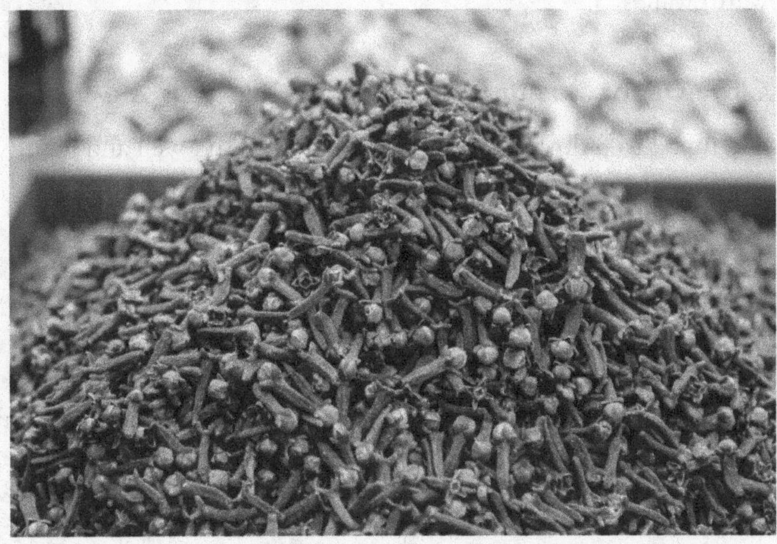

Clove-Based Mouthwash: Combine one cup vodka, 1 tablespoon whole cloves, 1 tablespoon cinnamon bark chips, 1 tablespoon fennel seed, 1 tablespoon anise seed and 1 tablespoon licorice root in a small glass jar, and seal the lid tightly. Leave the mixture as it is for two weeks; shake it daily to keep spices from settling. Once ready, strain the liquid and store it into a glass bottle. To use, dilute 1 tablespoon mouthwash in 1 cup water.

Cloves for Pedicuring (for Feet): Place 1 cup dried sage leaves and 1 teaspoon whole cloves into a coffee grinder, and process until finely ground. Now use this powder regularly on the feet before pedicuring. Just sprinkle the powder onto the feet and keep it there for sometime before soaking the feet in warm water.

Clove Oil for Moisturizing Dry Skin: Take your skin cream and mix 2 to 3 drops of pure clove oil to it. Mix well and gently massage on your skin. In order to fight the premature sign of ageing, apply clove oil on your face with the help of cotton ball twice a day.

Clove Oil for Beautiful Hair: For getting beautiful hair, just apply some clove oil on your scalp. It boosts blood circulation and helps to reduces hair fall and promotes hair growth. It also provides shine to dry and dull hair. You can also use equal parts of clove oil and olive oil as a great hair conditioner. Apply this mixture on your hair and wrap a warm towel around it. Let it stay for 20 minutes and then rinse it off with cold water.

Garlic as Natural Cosmetics

Garlic has antibacterial properties and hence helps to kill the bacteria causing acne and pimples. It also helps to reduce swelling and inflammation and improves blood circulation on the skin. Garlic can also work magic on lifeless hair. How to use garlic as a beauty aid on skin and hair is given below.

Garlic for Beautiful Hair: Rub sliced cloves of garlic on your scalp and then massage gently. After 15-20 minutes, wash off the hair with a mild shampoo. In addition to preventing hair loss, this treatment is also effective for removing dandruff.

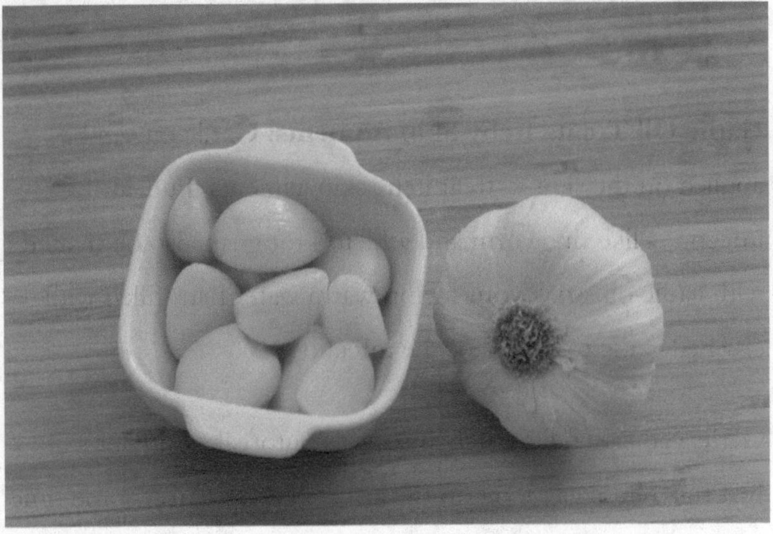

Garlic Clears Acne and Pimples: Just rub a sliced clove of garlic on the pimples, acne and other skin blemishes. Doing this treatment regularly will help to prevent the occurrence of pimples and acne.

Garlic Oil for Preventing Dandruff and Hair Loss: Garlic oil helps to prevent dandruff and hair loss. Massage your scalp thoroughly with garlic oil. Leave it overnight and rinse it off with cold water and shampoo the next day. This treatment helps to reduce hair fall and dandruff occurrence.

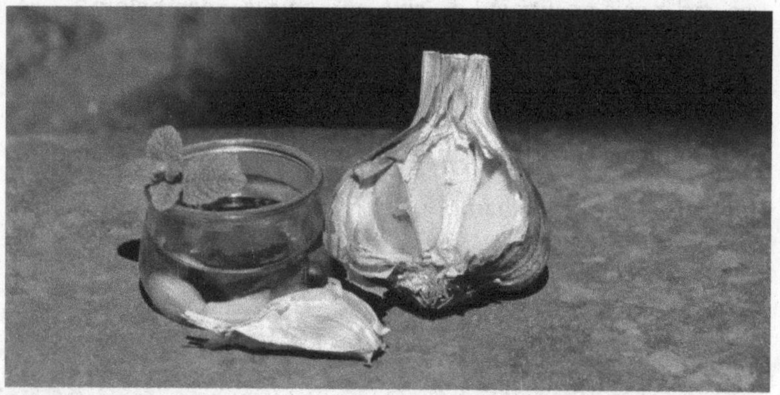

Garlic Oil Treats Itchy Skin Ailments: Garlic oil can be applied on the skin to treat itchy skin ailments. Fungal infections like ringworm and athlete's foot can also be treated with garlic oil. Soak your feet in warm water bath filled with crushed garlic to get rid of the infection.

Garlic can also relieve itchy psoriasis outbreaks on your skin. Just rub a little garlic oil on the affected areas. After some time wash it off and see the result for yourself.

Garlic for Memory and Brain Health: Research studies on garlic health benefits suggest that aged garlic extracts contain a high amount of an antioxidant called kyolic acid. This powerful antioxidant may help protect the brain from damage due to aging and diseases. This antioxidant may also help improve memory, concentration and focus in some people.

Garlic for Removing Dead Skin Cells: This treatment will exfoliate your skin and help remove dead skin cells that are blocking your skin pores. Mix 4 pureed cloves of garlic with 1 tablespoon of yogurt. Massage this paste into skin and leave it on for a few minutes. After that rinse it off with water. This treatment is very effective to remove dead skin cells.

Ginger Root As Natural Cosmetics

Do you know that even ginger has some beauty benefits? It contains powerful antioxidants properties that prevent free radical damage. Ginger has anti- aging benefits too. However, ginger-based natural cosmetics are not recommended for those whose skin is sensitive and allergic to this spice.

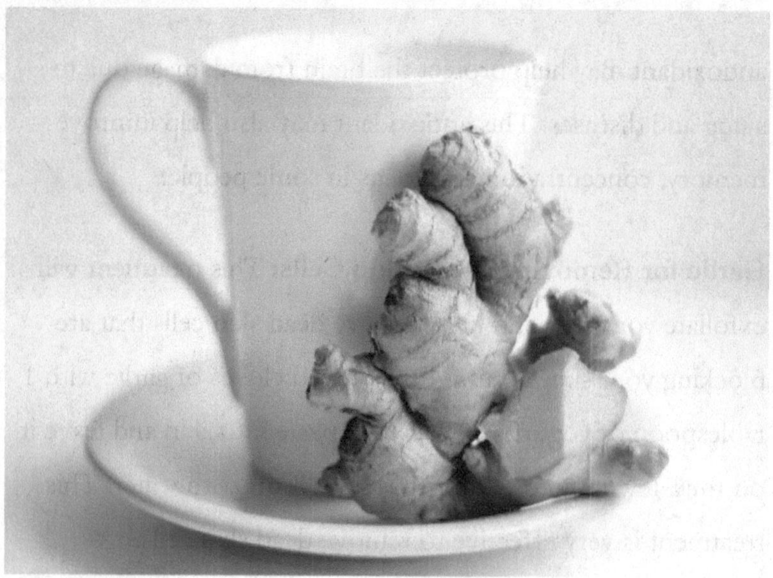

Ginger for Scars: Rub slices of fresh ginger onto the areas of your skin that are having scars, and let the ginger juice dry. After that, wash it off with cold water. Do this beauty treatment once or twice a day, every day and you should start to see the scars disappearing slowly and gradually within a couple of weeks. Within a few months, your scars will be undetectable and almost gone.

Ginger for Hair Growth: Ginger increases circulation to your scalp, which is essential for stimulating hair growth. Take equal parts of ginger oil and jojoba oil and massage it into your hair, concentrating on the scalp. Leave it for 30 minutes and then rinse it off with shampoo as usual.

Ginger Rejuvenates Skin: Both consuming ginger and applying it have major anti-aging benefits. It also evens skin tone. For this take equal parts of ginger powder, honey and lemon juice and mix the ingredients well to prepare a mask. Apply this mask on your skin and leave it for 30 minutes. Then rinse it off with cold water to reveal a radiant and glowing skin.

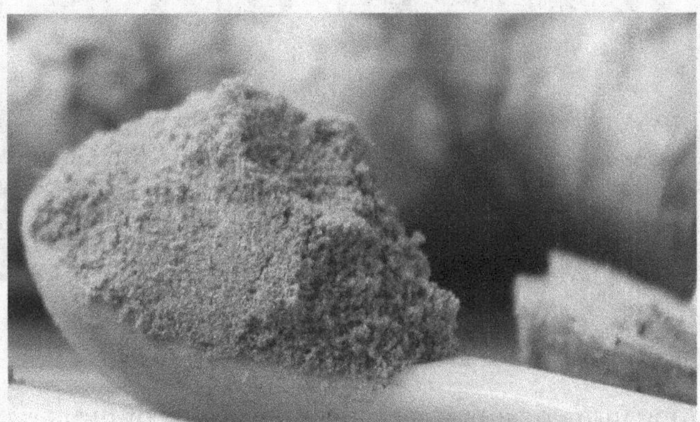

Ginger for Treating Dandruff: Ginger properties make it an excellent remedy for dandruff. Massage ginger oil or a mixture of two parts freshly grated ginger and three parts olive or sesame oil onto your scalp and let it set for 15-20 minutes. Do this treatment twice weekly for a few weeks for best results.

Turmeric As Natural Cosmetics

Turmeric is the most used and the most glorious spice in the beauty industry for its multiple benefits for skin and health. Turmeric has bleaching, antibacterial, antiseptic, and anti-inflammatory properties that help fight acne, pimple and other skin problems, brighten skin tone and reduce lines and wrinkles on the face. Let's see how turmeric can be used as a natural cosmetic as below:

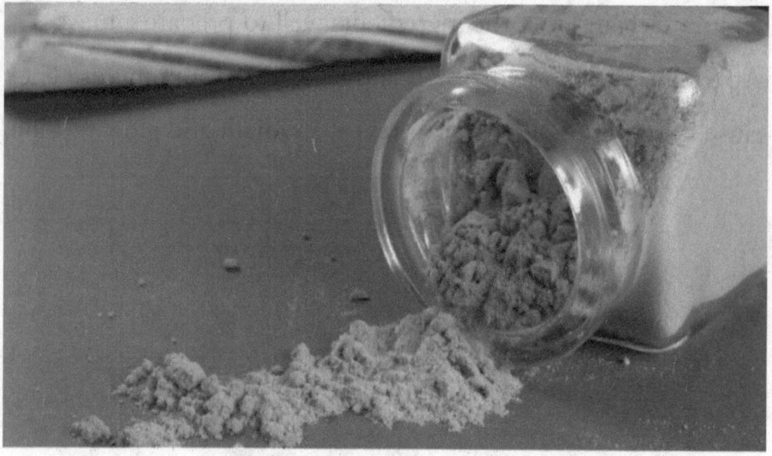

Turmeric Lotion for Bright Golden Complexion: For preparing turmeric lotion just add a few drops of turmeric essential oil to a cream or oil-based moisturizer and use it as you would use your regular moisturizer.

Turmeric as Facial Hair Remover: For removing your unwanted facial hair, prepare a turmeric-based cosmetic by combining ½ cup cold milk, ½ cup flour, 2 tablespoons of turmeric powder and 1 tablespoon sea salt. Mix them until it forms a sticky paste. Apply the paste to the area where you would like to stop the hair growth. Let the mask dry for some time. The mask will start to crumble off as it dries. After removing the mask, rinse the face with warm water and pat dry with a cloth.

Turmeric for Clear and Acne-Free Skin: Mix one tablespoon of raw honey with one teaspoon of turmeric powder. If you want you can add a few drops of lemon juice too. Mix the ingredients well until it becomes a thick paste and then apply this paste to skin. Rinse it off with warm water after 10-15 minutes.

Turmeric Night Serum: Mix 4 tablespoons of aloe vera gel with 10 drops of turmeric essential oil and 1 teaspoon argan oil. Apply the mixture to face before bed time. Wash it in the morning. Regular use of turmeric night serum will bless you with youthful-looking, wrinkle-free, blemish-free glowing skin.

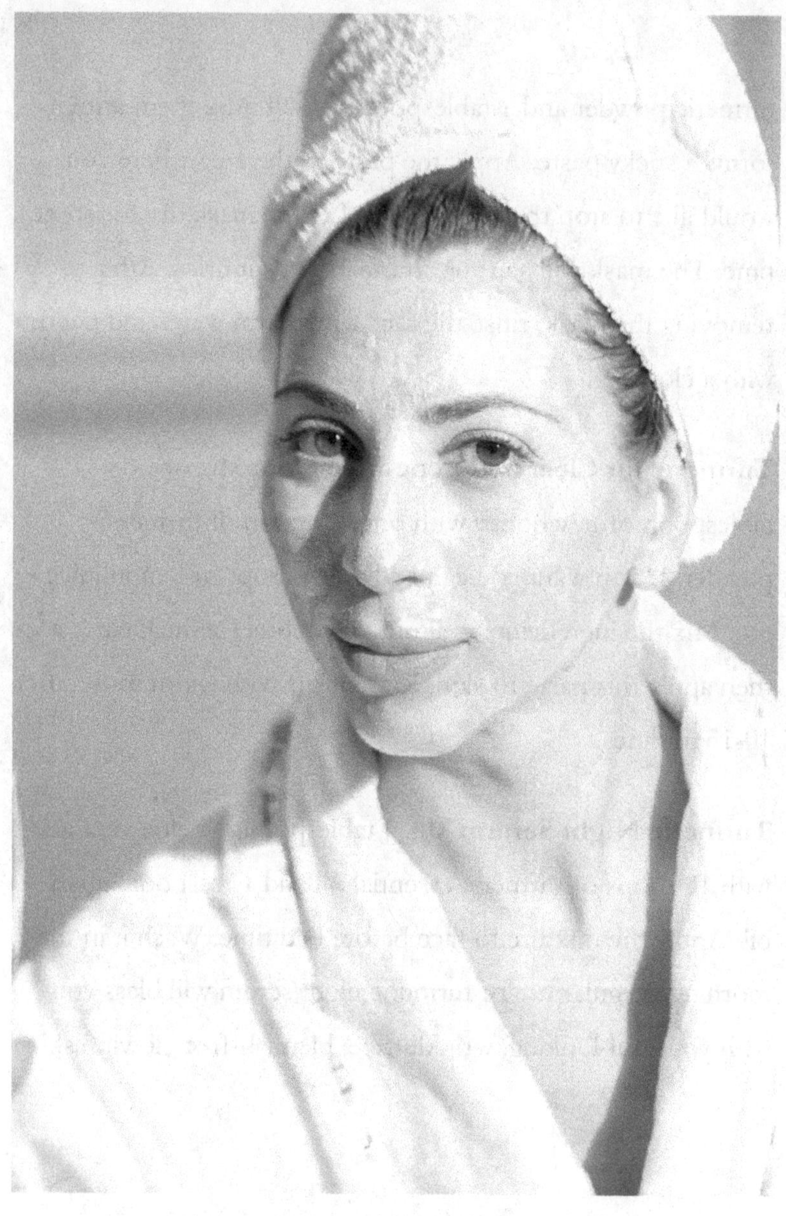

Turmeric Scrub for Removing Excess Oil from Face:
Using turmeric powder with gram flour as a natural scrub is good for all skin types and it is very gentle on the skin. It also removes excess oil from the skin. Mix turmeric powder with gram flour, and add a little water to make a paste. Apply this mixture on your skin using circular motion. Let it dry before washing it off with cold water.

Turmeric for Younger Looking Skin: Turmeric contains many antioxidants that can help make your skin look young and fresh. Mix equal parts of turmeric powder and olive oil properly. Use it on your face and neck. Let it stay a while and massage lightly to help stimulate the cells. Wash it off after half an hour to reveal supple skin.

Turmeric for Removing Stretch Marks: Mix equal parts of turmeric, saffron and lime juice. Apply the paste on the stretch marks and leave it for 15 minutes and then wash it off. Repeat this treatment every day for a few days or until you see that the marks are almost gone.

Turmeric for Brightening Dull Skin: Make a paste with turmeric powder, lemon juice and honey and apply it on your face and neck. Let it dry and then wash the face with lukewarm water. Regular use will make your skin bright and soft.

Curd and Yogurt as Natural Cosmetics

Yogurt is one of the most popular natural cosmetics that can be used for all skin types. You can use yogurt as a face cream or facial mask. Calcium present in the yogurt boosts new cells formation. Yoghurt is also good as a skin lotion when mixed with right ingredients. Let's see how to use curd/yogurt to enhance our beauty.

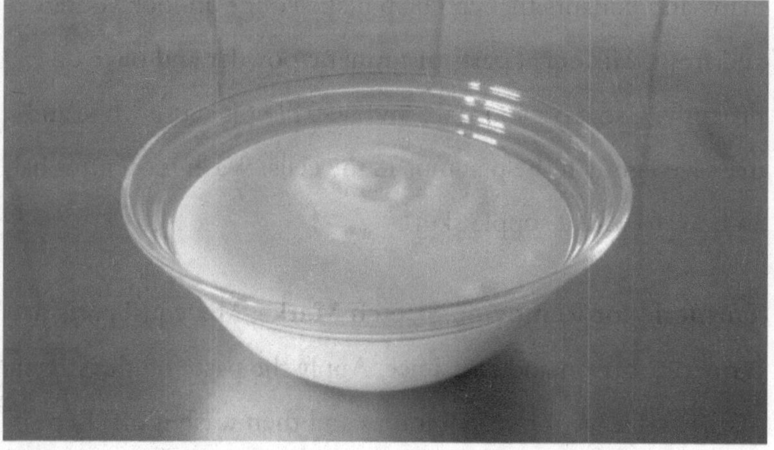

Yogurt as a Face Cleanser and Scrub: Mix two tablespoons of yogurt with one tablespoon of rice flour or oats. Apply this paste on your skin. Massage it in a circular motion to remove the dead skin cells as well as other impurities. Leave it for 10 minutes and then wash it off with water. This paste is both a cleanser and an exfoliator.

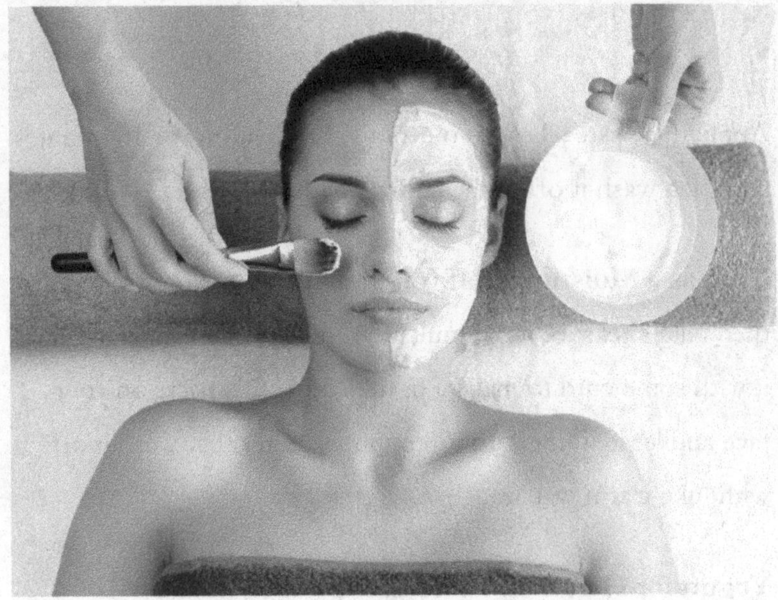

Yogurt Eliminates Dandruff: Just apply and massage some yogurt on your scalp and leave it on for 40 minutes. Then rinse it off with shampoo. Use this treatment once a week for a few weeks or until the dandruff is gone.

Curd as a Hair Conditioner: Take one cup of yogurt, an egg and some olive oil. Mix them well. Apply this mixture all over your hair and then put on a shower cap. Then wash it off thoroughly after half an hour. Use this treatment twice a month to keep your hair healthy.

Curd for Removing Sun Tan: Mix some curd with lemon juice and apply it all over your skin to effectively remove tan. You can also use orange peel powder with curd to form a paste that will remove tan and also add a glow to skin.

Apply this paste all over your body. Leave it on for 15 minutes and then wash it off in the shower with cold water.

Curd as a Moisturizer: If you want to use curd for oily skin, then take 2 teaspoons of multani mitti (Fuller's earth) and mix it with some curd to make a paste. Apply this paste on your face and let it sit there for 20 minutes. After that wash it off with luke warm water.

Yogurt for Hair Fall: Take half cup of yogurt and 3 tablespoons of ground fenugreek seeds. Make a paste. Apply the paste to your hair with the help of a brush. You can wash off the paste after an hour with the help of a mild shampoo.

Curd for Dark Circles: Curd can be used to remove your dark circles. Just dip a cotton ball in some yogurt and gently dab it under your eyes. Rinse it after 10 minutes. Do this treatment regularly until the dark circles are gone.

Yogurt for Treating Acne: Mix equal parts of gram flour and curd and make a smooth paste. Apply this paste on your face and wait for an hour. Then wash it off with water. Use this twice in a week to get clear and acne-free skin.

Ghee as a Natural Cosmetic

Ghee is considered to be a power food. Ghee act as healing agent for the body as it has good cholesterol and the fatty acids. Ghee can also be used as a natural cosmetic to make various face packs and skin and hair moisturizers. Let's see how to use ghee for better skin and hair care.

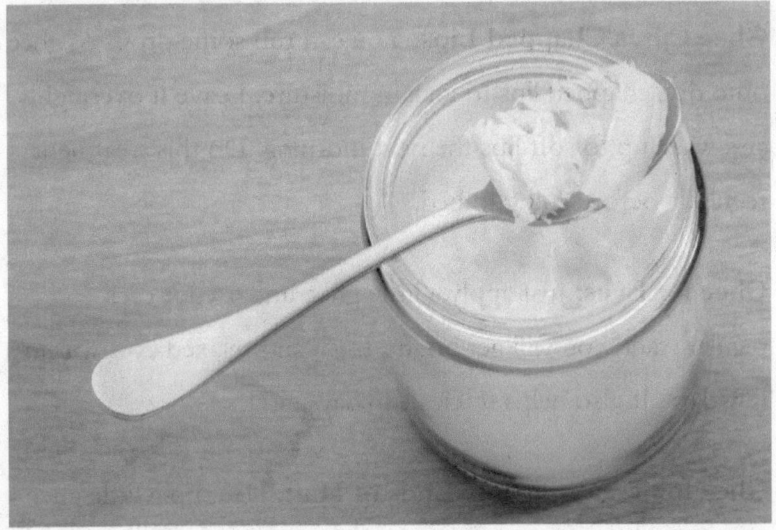

Ghee Moisturizes your Skin: Take equal parts of ghee and water and massage this solution on your face. Let it sit for 15 minutes and then wash it off with cold water. You will get soft and smooth skin instantly.

Ghee Hydrates Dry Skin: Before going for bath, just heat half a bowl of ghee and massage your entire body for 3-5 minutes. Then take your bath. It is the perfect way to hydrate your skin during winters.

Ghee for Bright Skin: Take equal parts of raw milk, ghee and gram flour. Make a smooth paste and apply it to your face and neck. Wash it off after 15-20 minutes.

Ghee Slows down Skin Aging: Massaging ghee on your skin on daily basis can beat ageing by many years.

Ghee Cures Chapped Lips: You can rub some drops of ghee onto dry, chapped lips to lock in moisture. Leave it overnight and wake up to soft lips the next morning. Do this treatment regularly before going to bed.

Ghee for Eyes: Just apply a little ghee under your eyes regularly and you will get bright, fresh and relaxed eyes within a few days. It also helps to clear up dark circles.

Ghee for Treating Split-Ends of Hair: Heat up a little ghee and apply it to the ends of your hair. Let it be there for an hour. Then wash it off with a mild shampoo. Do this process once a week for a few weeks for good results.

Ghee for Hair Growth: You can use ghee to promote your hair growth. Just massage your scalp with warm ghee mixed with equal parts of coconut oil. Then wash it off after an hour. It helps to nourish your scalp.

Milk and Milk Cream as Natural Cosmetics

Raw milk has many skin benefits. Milk can do wonders for your face and skin. Milk helps to nourish skin cells from deep within and also keeps skin moisturized all day. Let's go through the recipes of some milk-based natural cosmetics below:

Milk as a Skin Toner: Milk is a good skin toner for all the skin types. It makes the skin more elastic. Just add a few drops of lemon juice to raw milk. Mix well. If you have dry skin then you can add rose water too. Apply it on your face and neck and wait for 15 minutes. Later wash it off with water.

Milk as a Moisturizer: Add 2/3 tablespoon of gram flour to raw milk and mix well until it becomes a smooth paste. Now add few drops of raw honey and rose water and mix well again. Apply it on your face and neck. Wash it off with lukewarm water after 10 minutes.

Milk as a Skin Cleanser: Mix together 2 tablespoons of milk, a few drops of lemon juice and 2 tablespoons of cucumber juice. Apply it on your face and neck by using a cotton ball. Wait for 8-10 minutes and then wash it off with water. You will get clear and bright skin instantly.

Milk Treats Dry Skin: Mix 2 tablespoons of raw milk and 1 tablespoon honey. Apply this mixture on your face and neck with a cotton ball and leave it for 15-20 minutes. Then wash it off with water to get clean, moisturized skin.

Milk Soothes Sunburn: Use a cotton ball dipped in cold milk to apply milk on sun-burn areas. This treatment soothes and relieves sunburns. Milk creates a thin protein film over the affected areas and thus helps to protect our skin and also cools down burning sensations.

Milk for Feet and Heels: This homemade foot soak will help to soften cracked heels and relax your feet. It also helps to relieve any foot tension and pain. Take 2 cups of warm milk and 4 cups of warm water in a tub. Soak your feet and rub your cracked heels with pumice stone and dry them with a towel. After this treatment your feet will feel super soft and moisturized.

Milk Treats Dry Scalp: Milk gives a soothing effect on the scalp and promote hair texture and luster. To treat a dry scalp with milk, mix ½ cup milk with ¼ cup honey and apply this directly on your scalp. Put a shower cap and leave it on for 2 hours. Then wash it off with a mild shampoo.

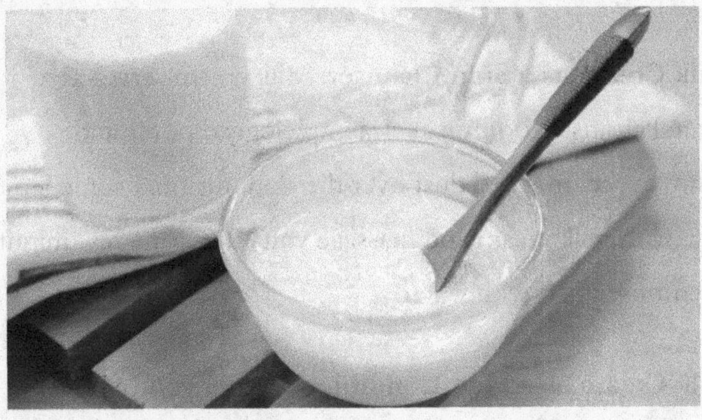

Milk Cream Removes Dark Spots: Just massage your face and neck with some milk cream gently and softly for 15-20 minutes and then rinse it off with luke warm water. This facial treatment helps to get rid of dead skin cells which cause dark spots on the face.

Milk Cream for Treating Dry Skin and for Getting Glowing Skin: Mix one tablespoon of milk cream with one tablespoon of gram flour and make a paste. Apply this paste on your face and neck and leave it for 20 minutes. Then rinse it off with cold water. Do this twice or thrice every week for better results.

Milk Cream Scrub for Removing Dead Skin: Just mix some oats with milk cream and use it as a scrub. Rub this mixture to your skin that has dead skin cells like elbow, knee, neck, arm and legs. Rub it gently for 5-10 minutes and wash it off with cold water. For best results, do this treatment twice every week.

Milk Cream as a Skin Cleanser: Milk cream serves as a natural cleanser too. It can clean up clogged pores and removes accumulated dust over the skin. Just mix some lemon juice with milk cream and massage your skin for a few minutes. Then rinse it off with water.

Milk Cream as a Hair Conditioner: After you've done shampooing hair, apply milk cream on your hair the same way you use a hair conditioner. After conditioning the hair with milk cream, rinse it off thoroughly. This treatment helps to condition the dry hair.

Milk Cream for Removing Dark Circles: Milk cream can also help in reducing darkness around your eyes. Mix one tablespoon of milk cream with one tablespoon of castor oil. Apply the mixture around the eyes very gently. Leave it on for 15-20 minutes and rinse off with lukewarm water. This treatment reduces both puffiness and darkness around the eyes.

Milk Cream for Preventing Premature Ageing: If you don't want prematurely aging skin, then resort to milk cream beauty treatment. Simply mix milk cream with a pinch of turmeric powder and apply it on your face. Wait for 15 minutes and then wash it with lukewarm water. Do the treatment regularly.

Milk Powder As A Natural Cosmetic

Milk powder acts as a cleanser. It gives youthful glow to your skin. It has lactic acid, which lightens and smoothens the skin. It hydrates your skin too. Milk powder face packs help in removing blackheads as well as whiteheads. Hence, it gives a healthy and glowing skin. It also protects your skin from sunburn. It has endless numbers of benefits. Let's look at the recipes of some of the milk powder - based cosmetics given below.

Milk Powder for Lighter Skin: For getting a brighter and lighter skin tone, all you need is 2 tablespoons of fresh orange juice, 1 tablespoon of oatmeal powder and 1 tablespoon of milk powder. Take a bowl and mix all these ingredients to form a paste. Apply this paste on your face. Keep it on for 20 minutes and then wash it off with cold water. Within a week of regular use, your skin should shine bright like a diamond.

Milk Powder for Treating Pigmentation: Take 2 tablespoons of milk powder, 2 tablespoons of yogurt and half a lemon's juice. Mix them to form a thick paste. Soak a towel in warm water and steam your face to open your pores. Now apply the paste to your face and leave it for 20 minutes. Then wash it off with water. Repeat this treatment every third day for a few weeks for getting the desired results.

Milk Powder for Treating Pimples: Take 1 teaspoon of

turmeric powder, 1 teaspoon of milk powder and 1 tablespoon of honey. Mix them well and apply evenly on your face. Let it dry for some time and then wash it off with lukewarm water. Do this process twice a week to get rid of acne and its blemishes.

Milk Powder for Removing Oil from Skin: For this take equal parts of fuller's earth (multani mitti) and milk powder. Mix both the ingredients well to make a smooth paste by using some rose water. Apply it on your face evenly and let it dry thoroughly. Wash it off with lukewarm water to get fresher skin instantly.

Milk Powder for Treating Dry Skin: Mash a ripe banana fruit. Mix it with 1 tablespoon of milk powder. Now apply this paste on your face and leave it on for 20 minutes. Then wash your face with normal water. This simple remedy not only treats dry skin but also makes your skin tone bright.

Milk Powder for Removing Sun Tan: For treating suntan, milk powder is the best natural remedy. Take half of a ripe tomato fruit and blend it in a blender to form a paste. Now add 2 tablespoons of milk powder to it. Mix it well and apply this paste on the areas where is sun burn. Leave it on for 30 minutes. Later, wash it off your skin with normal water.

Mustard Oil as a Natural Cosmetic

Mustard oil has wonderful cosmetic properties and therefore it is also used as a beauty remedy to encourage hair growth, provide nourishment to skin, oral health and so on. There are many ways of using mustard oil on your skin and hair. Some popular recipes are discussed below.

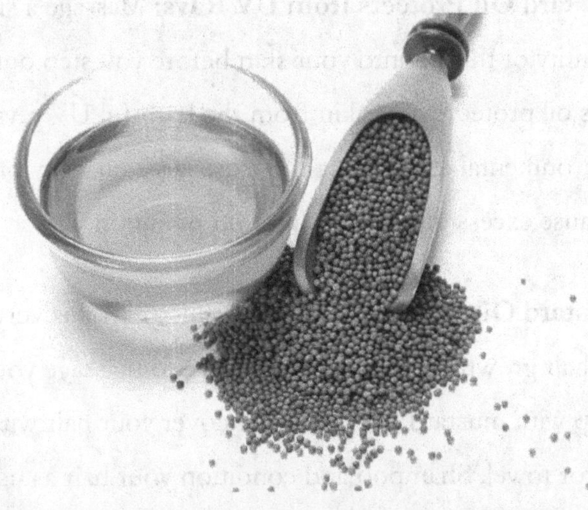

Mustard Oil Heals Chapped Lips: Do you have chapped lips? Don't worry. Just apply two or three drops of mustard oil in your navel every night before going for sleep. As long as you do this every night, you should never have to worry about having chapped lips over again.

Mustard Oil Whitens Teeth: Take ½ teaspoon of mustard oil, 1 teaspoon of turmeric powder and ½ teaspoon of salt. Mix all the ingredients. You can rub this mixture on your teeth and gums twice a day. It will promote healthy teeth.

Mustard Oil Removes Sun Tan and Dark Spots and Lightens The Skin Tone: Take equal parts of mustard oil and coconut oil. Mix them and massage it on your skin every day. After 15 minutes wash it off. Use it regularly for the desired results.

Mustard Oil Protects from UV Rays: Massage a small quantity of this oil into your skin before you step outdoors. This oil protects your skin from the harmful UV rays and environmental toxins. But don't use large quantity of this oil because excess oil attracts dust and pollution.

Mustard Oil for Hair Growth: Using this oil is very beneficial for hair growth. You just simply have to massage your hair and scalp with mustard oil. After that cover your hair with a shower cap or towel. Shampoo and condition your hair as usual after 3 hours. After a few treatments, you will see great results. It also helps to prevent premature greying of hair if used regularly.

Mustard Oil for Treating Dandruff and Itchy Scalp: Mix equal amounts of mustard oil and coconut oil and massage into the hair. Now cover your hair with a towel. Leave it as such for 2 hours. Wash it off with a mild shampoo. Do this a few times a week and watch your dandruff disappears slowly.

Olive Oil As A Natural Cosmetic

Olive oil is full of anti-aging antioxidants which help in promoting health of hair, skin and nails. Olive oil has lots of medicinal properties as well. Hydrating properties of olive oil keep your skin hydrated always. Some of the uses of olive oil on skin and hair is given below.

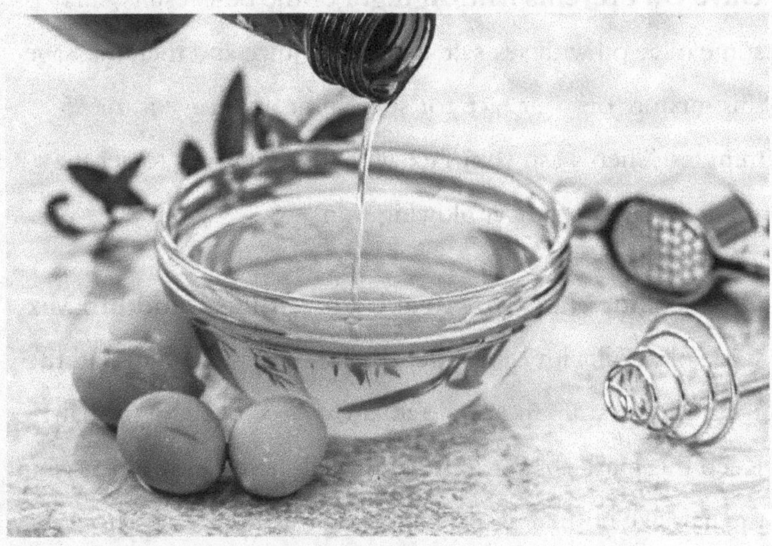

Olive Oil as a Pre-Shampoo Hair Treatment: First of all warm the olive oil. Then apply it gently to the ends of hair and scalp. Leave it for 20 minutes and then wash it off with the help of a shampoo.

Olive Oil Lip Scrub: Combine sugar with a teaspoon of olive oil for a chapped lip fix. You can also add lemon juice for its exfoliating properties.

Olive Oil for Cracked Heels: Split, rough heels need moisture to heal. After exfoliating with pumice stone, apply olive oil to feet. Put on socks to lock in the hydrating treatment as you sleep.

Olive Oil Prevents Anti-Aging: For the best results, mix some olive oil with sea salt and lemon juice and then massage this mixture on your face for some time and leave it for 15 minutes. Then wash your face with normal water to get the shinier and the younger glowing skin.

Olive Oil for Hair Growth and Preventing Dandruff: Mix some olive oil with egg white, yogurt and lemon juice and then apply on the scalp to get the advantages of olive oil for hair. Keep this mask for 20-25 minutes and then remove by washing the hair like normal. Repeat applying this hair mask once or twice a week to get the complete freedom from dandruff.

Olive Oil for Nail Health: Your nails need as much attention as your skin. For getting healthy nails, simply dip a cotton ball in 2-3 tablespoons of olive oil and dab it on your nails. Olive oil very helpful for your dry brittle nails.

Pulses As A Natural Cosmetic

Pulses especially, Bengal gram and green gram are packed with proteins and minerals that can help to get a glowing skin. It also does wonders for hair. Some of the popular recipes of pulses-based cosmetics are given below:

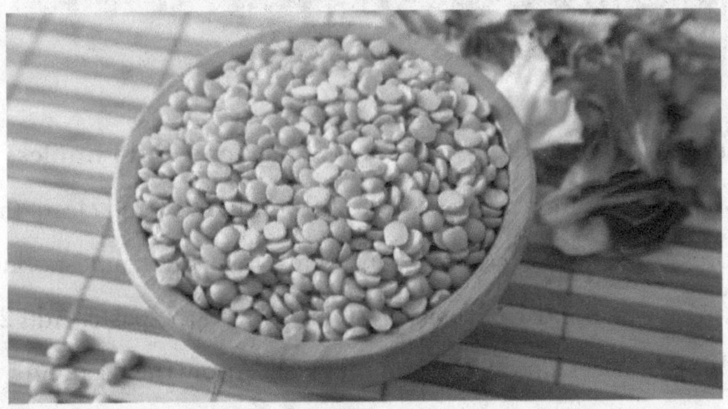

Bengal Gram and Green Gram Exfoliate Your Skin: Gram flour can be very effective scrub in removing dirt, stains and dead skin cells from the skin. Take a small cup of gram flour. Now add 2 tablespoons of milk and 2 tablespoons of ghee or melted butter to the paste and mix them well. Apply the paste on your face. Leave it for 30 minutes. Then wash it off with lukewarm water. Follow this thrice a week to remove dead skin cells.

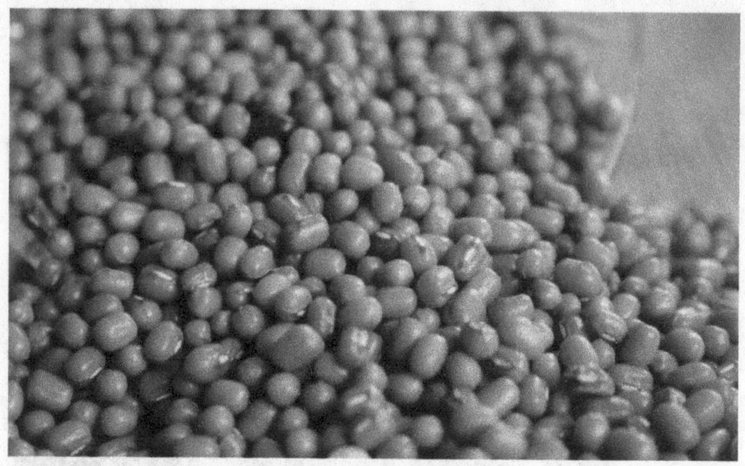

Bengal Gram and Green Gram Treat Acne and Pimples:
Gram flour removes the excess oil from the face and clears the pores. Take a small cup of gram flour. Now add 2 tablespoons of rose water and 1 tablespoon of glycerin to the paste. Add 2 tablespoons of almond oil and mix well. Apply the paste on your face. Let it dry for 15-20 minutes and then wash it with cold water. Apply this every alternate day for the better results.

Bengal Gram Face Mask for Skin Glow: If you have dull and uneven skin tone, then this bengal gram face mask is beneficial for you. Soak ¼ cup of bengal gram and 8-9 almonds overnight. Grind them in to paste next morning. Apply it on your face. Wait for 20 minutes. Then wash it off with cold water. Do this treatment thrice a week for the better results.

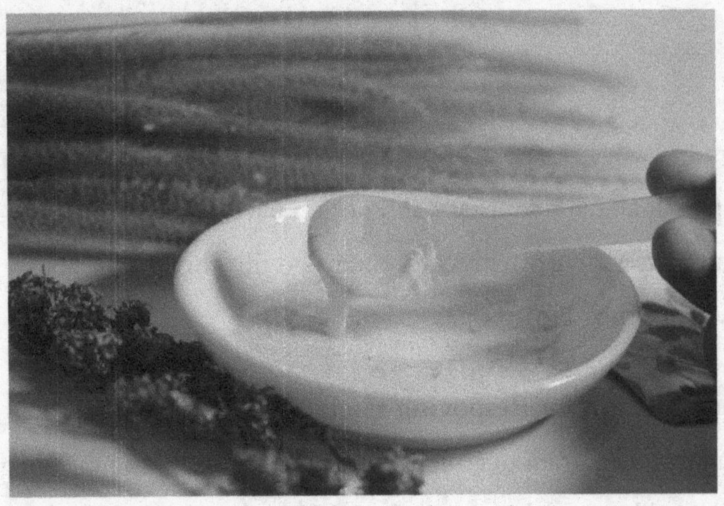

Bengal Gram and Green gram Removes Sun Tan and Heals Sunburn: Gram flour has cooling effect on skin which helps in healing sunburns. Take one small cup of gram flour. Now add 3 tablespoons of curd and mix well. Apply it on your face and sunburn area. Leave it for 15 minutes. Then wash it off with cold water. Do this treatment every alternate day for the better results.

Gram Flour for Dry and Fizzy Hair: This recipe is beneficial for dry brittle hair. It will also condition your hair and give it a shiny look. Take half cup gram flour. Now add 1 tablespoon of curd into it. Apply this on your hair. Leave it for 30 minutes and then wash it off with mild shampoo. Use this once a week and see the results.

Green Gram for Dry Skin: Soak two tablespoons of green gram overnight in some milk. Grind the same in the morning.

Apply it all over your face and neck. Leave it for 20 minutes and then wash off with cold water. Do this thrice a week to hydrate your skin.

Green Gram for Removing Facial Hair: For this soak half cup of green gram overnight and make a paste in the morning. Now add two tablespoons of sandalwood powder and two tablespoons of orange peel powder to the paste. Now make a fine paste by using some milk. Apply it on your face and scrub it in circular motion to deal with dry skin. Then wash off with cold water. Do this treatment thrice a week to get the desired results.

Green Gram Removes Sun Tan: For removing your sun tan soak ¼ cup of green gram in water overnight. Make a fine paste in the morning. Now add two tablespoons of yogurt and apply this paste on your affected area. Let it sit there for 10 minutes. Then wash it off with cold water. Use this mixture every alternate day for getting the desired results.

Rice Water as a Natural Cosmetic

Rice water -the water left over after you cook rice-makes our hair strong and beautiful. Today, rice water is very popular as a natural cosmetic as it contains substances that help protect and repair your skin. It helps to soothe and tone your skin and improve different skin conditions. For making rice water just soak uncooked rice overnight in some water. Strain the water in the morning and your rice water is ready. Now let us see below the recipes of some popular rice water-based cosmetics.

Rice Water for Promoting Hair Growth: Apply the rice water to your hair from the roots to the ends and leave it on for at least 10 minutes. Then rinse it off with a mild shampoo. This treatment decreases hair fall and promotes hair growth. This treatment is also beneficial for curing dandruff and removing lice-infestation from the hair. Use the treatment thrice a week for the desired results.

Rice Water as a Facial Cleanser and Skin Toner: Put a small amount of rice water on a cotton ball and gently dab it on your face and neck as a toner. Clean it by massaging into your skin. Rinse it off after some time.

Rice Water as a Body Scrub: Add some salt and essential oil in to rice water and use it as a scrubber. Gently rub your body by using this scrub and after 10 minutes wash it off with water.

Rice water Soothes Sunburn: Rice water is helpful in soothing sunburn, redness and itching problems. Just simply apply rice water on affected areas by using a cotton ball. Leave it for some time. Then wash it off with cold water.

Rice Water Hand Soak: Rice water helps to reduce dryness and dark spots on hands. It gives a youthful glow and suppleness to hands. Take some amount of rice water in a bowl. Now add some drops of essential oil such as lavender oil, sandalwood oil or any other suitable essential oil to it. Now soak your hands in this water for at least 15 minutes. Then rinse it off with cold water. After that apply some moisturizer if you desire.

Coffee As A Natural Cosmetic

Coffee powder can also work wonders on your skin and it will effectively smoothen, protect and stimulate the skin. Please below some recipes of coffee-based natural cosmetics.

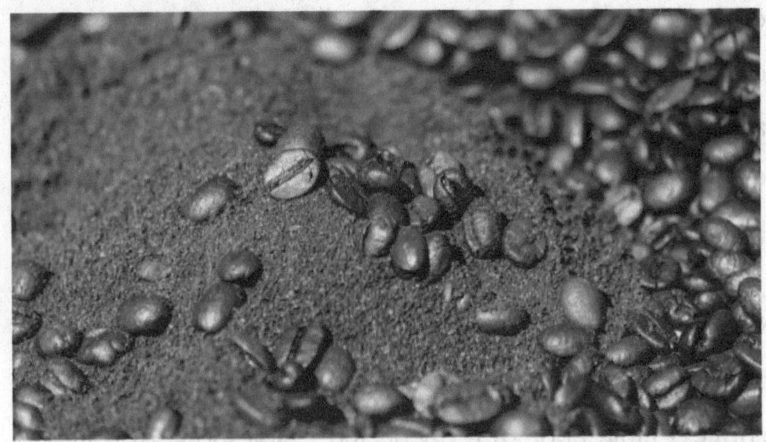

Coffee for Removing Dark Circles under the Eyes: If you have dark circles around the eyes, then use this coffee-based under-eye pack. Mix two tablespoons of coffee powder with one tablespoon of coconut oil. Mix well and apply this paste under your eyes. Leave it for 20 minutes and wash if off with water and a face wash. This coffee mask will reduce the puffiness and dark circles around the eyes.

Coffee Skin Scrub: To make it, combine 1 tablespoon of ground coffee, 2 tablespoons of brown sugar and 1 tablespoon of olive oil. Mix all the ingredients well to make a cream. Now gently massage this cream all over your face and neck. Let it sit for 30 minutes and then wash it off with warm water. This scrub removes dead skin cells and impurities from your skin and makes your face smoother and cleaner.

Coffee Face Mask for Skin Brightening: For making this face mask, combine 1 tablespoon of coffee powder, 1 teaspoon of turmeric powder, 1 tablespoon of cold milk and 2-3 strands of saffron. Mix the ingredients well and make a paste. Apply it all over your face and neck. Let it dry for 40 minutes and then wash it off with cold water. This beauty treatment will make your skin radiant and bright.

Coffee Mask for Clear Skin Tone: This mask is very helpful to get a clear and flawless glowing skin. Take 1 tablespoon of coffee, 1 tablespoon of turmeric and 1 tablespoon of yogurt. Mix them well. Apply it on your face in downward motion and let it sit there for 20 minutes. Then rinse it off with normal water. This face mask will eliminate the dead cells from your face and rejuvenates it. Apply it twice a week for the better results.

Coffee Face Mask for Glowing and Smooth Skin: Mix one tablespoon of coffee powder and one tablespoon of honey. Mix them into a paste. Apply this paste on your face in downward motion and sit relaxed for 15-20 minutes. Then wash it off with lukewarm water. This mask tightens the skin cells and gives a healthy glowing skin.

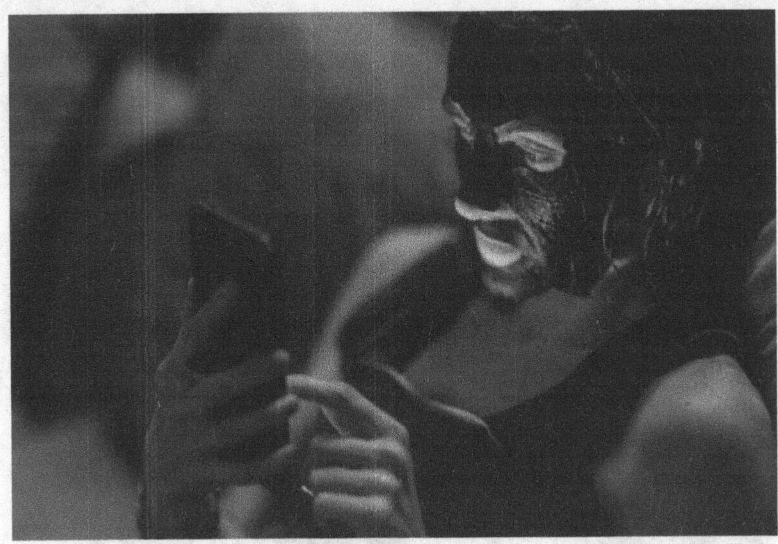

Coffee Face Mask for Removing Excess Oil from Skin:
Mix one tablespoon of coffee powder and one tablespoon of lemon juice. Mix well. Apply this paste on your face and neck and wait for 15 minutes. Then rinse off with normal water. Use this treatment once a week to get an oil-free and glowing skin.

Coffee Powder for Pedicuring Feet: Take 1 cup of coconut oil, ½ cup of coffee powder and 2 tablespoons of vanilla extract in a bowl and mix them well. Now soak your feet in a tub of warm soapy water. Use this paste to scrub your feet in a circular motion. Then wash your feet and pat dry.

Eggs as Natural Cosmetics

Every part of egg such as egg white, egg yolk and even egg shell can be used as natural cosmetics. Eggs are commonly used for hair treatment. It promotes hair growth and makes it silky and shiny. Popular recipes of some egg-based natural cosmetics are given below:

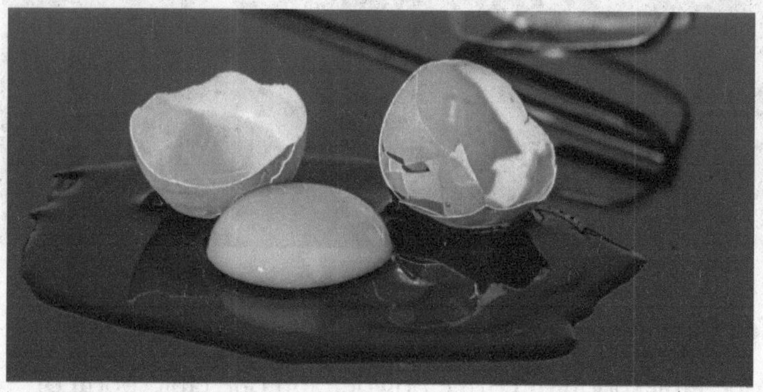

Egg White for Soothing Burns and Removing Scars: Egg whites not only help in healing burns but also remove scars. Apply egg whites on affected skin areas and wait for 10-15 minutes. Then rinse it off with cold water.

Egg Yolk for Thicker Eyebrows: To get lush eyebrows, beat one egg yolk. Now dip a cotton ball in it and apply on your eyebrows. Wait for 15-20 minutes and then wash it off with cold water. Do this treatment for a few weeks on regular basis for getting the desired results.

Egg White for Tightening the Skin Pores: Take egg white

of one egg. Now add 1 tablespoon of lemon juice, 2 tablespoons of oatmeal and 1 shredded tomato. Blend all the ingredients in a blender and make a thick paste. Now apply this paste on your face and leave it for 10 minutes. Then rinse it off with warm water. Use this treatment twice a week to get the desired results.

Egg Yolk for Nails: Take a shallow bowl. Pour egg yolk of one or two large eggs. Now soak your palms in the egg yolk and wash after half an hour or more. This is a good nail cuticle treatment.

Egg White for Hair Health: Crack two eggs and take egg white only. Now add 1 tablespoon of olive oil in this egg white and mix well. Now apply this mixture on your dry hair but not on your scalp. Wait for 10 minutes and then wash it off with a mild shampoo. This hair treatment will make your hair silky and shiny.

Egg Yolk for Thick Hair: Take egg yolk according to the length of your hair. Beat them well. Then apply this egg yolk on your scalp and hair. Wait for half an hour. Then wash it off with a shampoo and luke warm water. This is a good treatment for thin hair. This protects our hair from any further hair damage. Do this treatment twice a week for the better results.

Eggs for Preventing Hair Fall: Beat one egg and add 3-4 tablespoons of curd and 1 tablespoon of lemon juice to it. Mix them well and make a paste. Now apply the mask on your scalp with the help of a brush. Let it stay there for about an hour. Then rinse it off with a shampoo. This mask not only strengthens weak hair but also gets rid of dandruff.

Eggs for Treating Dry Skin: Beat one egg and add ½ tablespoon of honey to it. Mix both the ingredients well and then apply it on your face and neck. Let it dry. Then wash it off with lukewarm water. This beauty treatment will moisturize your skin immediately.

Egg White for Removing Eye Puffiness: For puffy eyes just apply egg white under your eyes by using a cotton ball. Wait for 10 minutes and then wash it off. Do this treatment daily for the better results.

Honey and Beeswax as Natural Cosmetics

Honey has antifungal and antibacterial properties. Honey is very helpful in reducing dandruff. Honey is also recommended to apply on sun-burned area for faster healing. Honey also helps to make our hair strong, silky and shiny. There are many ways to use honey as natural cosmetics. Some of the recipes are stated below.

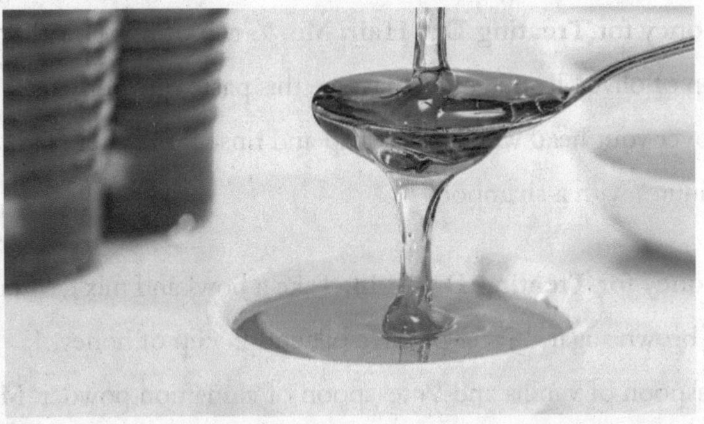

Honey for Treating Dandruff: Take honey and massage it on your scalp. Cover your hair with shower cap and leave it on for 3 hours. Then wash it off. Do this treatment daily for 2-3 weeks for better results.

Honey Eyelash Balm for Beautiful Eyelashes: For making your eyelashes more thick and beautiful you can use honey. Take 1 tablespoon of honey and 3 tablespoons of castor oil in a bowl. Cover it for a week until it becomes a smooth paste. After that you can use it daily on your eyelashes before going to bed. Do this treatment regularly until you see the difference in the growth of your eyelashes.

Honey for Treating Sunburn: For treating your sunburn just mix 1 teaspoon of honey, 1 teaspoon of olive oil and ¼ teaspoon of lemon juice. Mix the ingredients well and apply it on your sun-burned area. Wait for 10 minutes. Then wash it off with cold water.

Honey for Treating Dry Hair: Mix ½ cup of honey with ¼ cup of olive oil and gently massage this paste on your hair. Cover your head with shower cap and rinse it off after 30 minutes with a shampoo.

Honey for Treating Dry Skin: Take a bowl and mix 2 ¼ cup of brown sugar, ½ cup of olive oil, and ¼ cup of honey, 1 teaspoon of vanilla and ¼ teaspoon of cinnamon powder. Mix all the ingredients well. Store the mixture in an airtight container. You can use this scrub on your skin whenever you need.

Beeswax for Waxing and Removal of Unwanted Hair: Beeswax is a popular natural cosmetic used for removing unwanted hair. Take the required quantity of beeswax (according to the amount of hair you want to remove) in a bowl and melt it completely by using a double boiler. Take the melted beeswax out and place it at room temperature to cool down. Then apply it directly on the hair you want to remove by applying it in the direction of hair growth. Then let it dry. The beeswax will dry within seconds. Now it's time to remove the wax along with the hair. For this, just pull out the dried wax in the opposite direction of the hair growth. All unwanted hair is removed instantly.

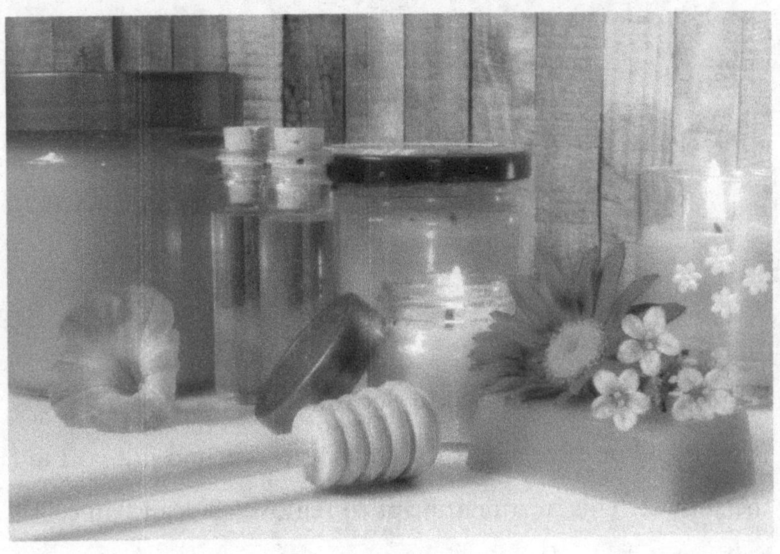

Sugar as a Natural Cosmetic

Sugar is very helpful for making a natural skin scrub. Sugar-based skin scrub can be used for getting a clear complexion. It helps to lighten the dark spots and suntan on the facial skin. Let's find out the several ways of using sugar as a natural cosmetic.

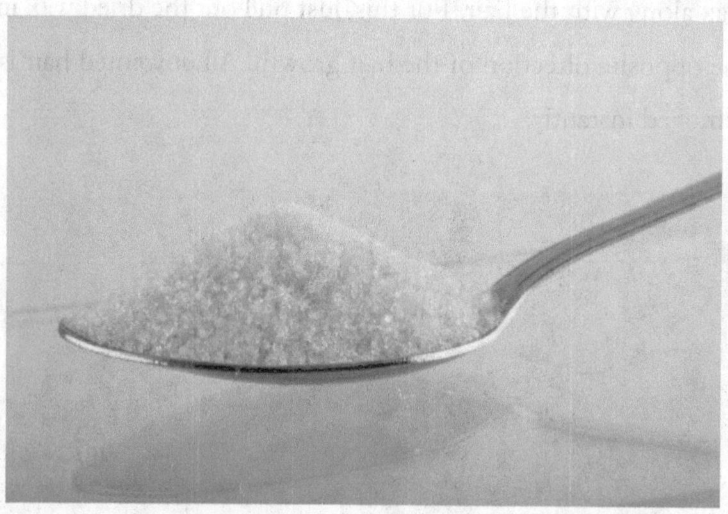

Sugar-Based Exfoliate Skin Scrub: Mix sugar with oil (almond oil or olive oil). Rub gently onto skin and rinse off in the shower. This treatment helps to remove all dead skin cells and make our body soft, supple and smooth.

Sugar Makes Your Lipstick Last: You can also use sugar to extend the wearing time of your lipstick. After applying your lipstick, simply sprinkle sugar powder on your lips.

Sugar for Smooth Lips: To nourish your dry lips, simply mix equal amount of sugar and olive oil to form a paste. Apply the mixture on your lips and let it sit for 1 minute. After that, wipe it off with a cloth. That's all. You will get your soft and smooth lips.

Sugar Scrub for Removing Sun Tan and Dark Spots: For making this scrub, take 2 tablespoons of sugar and juice of 4 limes. Massage this scrub on your face until sugar gets dissolved. Then wash it off with warm water. This scrub is very helpful for clearing dark spots and sun tan. Do this treatment regularly for getting good results.

Sugar Scrub for Getting Clear Skin Complexion: Mix equal parts of honey and sugar and massage it on your face and neck. Wait for 10 minutes and then wash it off with water. This treatment helps to remove all dead skin cells and leaves you with a clear complexion.

Sugar for Pedicuring Feet: Take the required quantity of sugar and add some quantity of peppermint oil. Now scrub this mixture on your feet for 2-5 minutes. Then wash it off. This treatment helps to remove dead cells from your feet.

Brown Sugar Scrub for Manicuring Hands: If you want gorgeous-looking hands, then take 1 cup of brown sugar and 1/3 cups of olive oil. Mix the ingredients well to make the paste and scrub the same on your hands for some time. Then wash it off. This treatment gives your hands a youthful and fresh look. This sugar scrub treatment may be given to your face and legs as well.

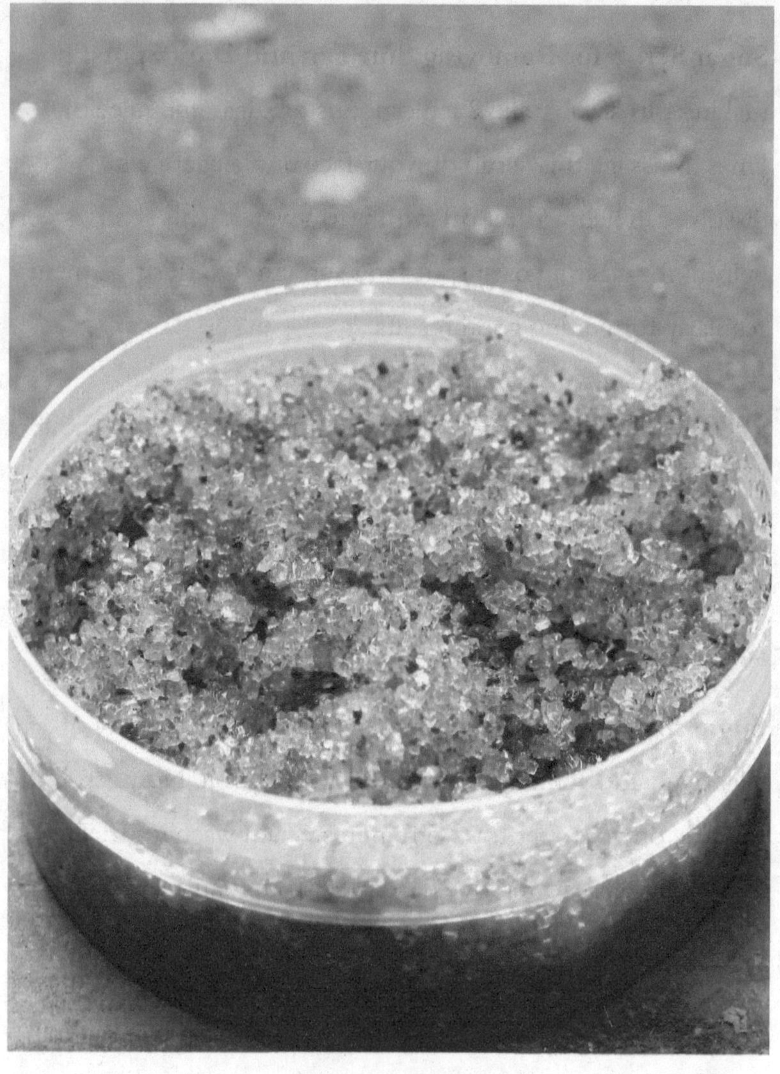

Tea as a Natural Cosmetic

The beauty and health benefits of drinking green tea, applying tea bags and tea leaves on your skin and hair are plenty. Now let us look at the various ways of using tea as a natural cosmetic as described below:

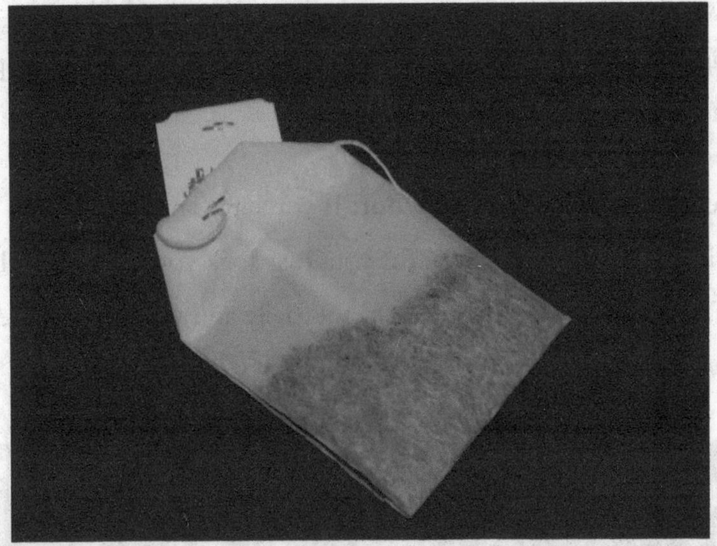

Tea Bags for Removing Puffy Eyes and Dark Circles: Just wet two tea bags and place them directly on your eyes. Keep it there for at least 10 minutes. Do this treatment daily for getting rid of dark circles and puffiness around the eyes.

Tea is Beneficial for Soothing Sun-burn: Soak some tea in a pan with water. Keep it overnight. Now dip a towel in this tea water and apply it on the affected areas. Keep the towel in place for at least 30 minutes. You can use wet tea bags for treating sun-burns on your face.

Tea Leaves and Tea Dust as a Scrubber: Massage the same on your face in circular motion for some minutes. Then wash your face with water. Your skin will feel smooth and soft. You can use used tea dust also for this treatment.

Tea for Chapped Lips: For fixing your chapped lips, take a green tea bag and soak it in warm water. Now apply this tea bag on your lips. Wait for 10 minutes. This will hydrate the lips and thus fix the chapped lips.

Tea for Removing Feet Odor: If you have smelly feet then this treatment is beneficial for you. Just soak your feet in a tub of tea water for 20 minutes. Do this daily and your feet will feel awesome.

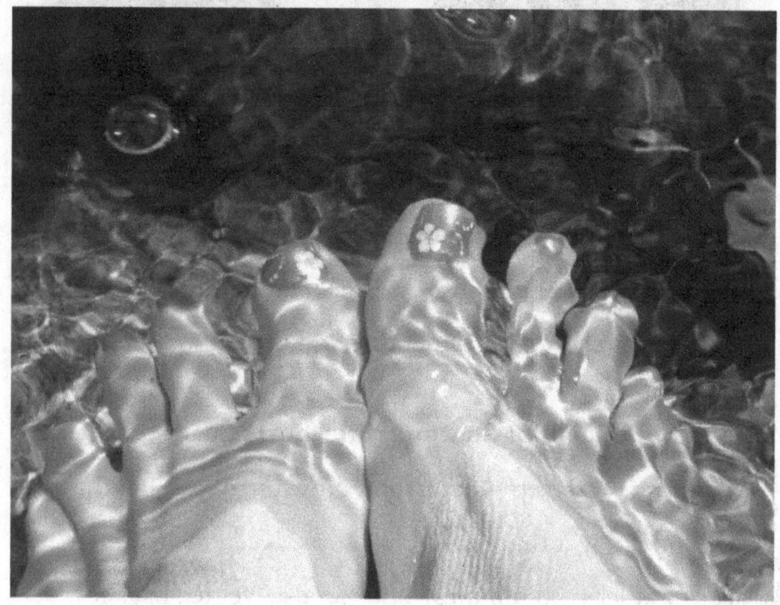

Tea Hair Cleanser: You can use black tea for making an amazing cleanser for hair. In order to stop your tresses from shedding, soak some black tea in warm water. Let it cool and store the same in the spray bottle. Spray it into your hair daily before going to bed. It cleanses your scalp and makes your hair look lustrous.

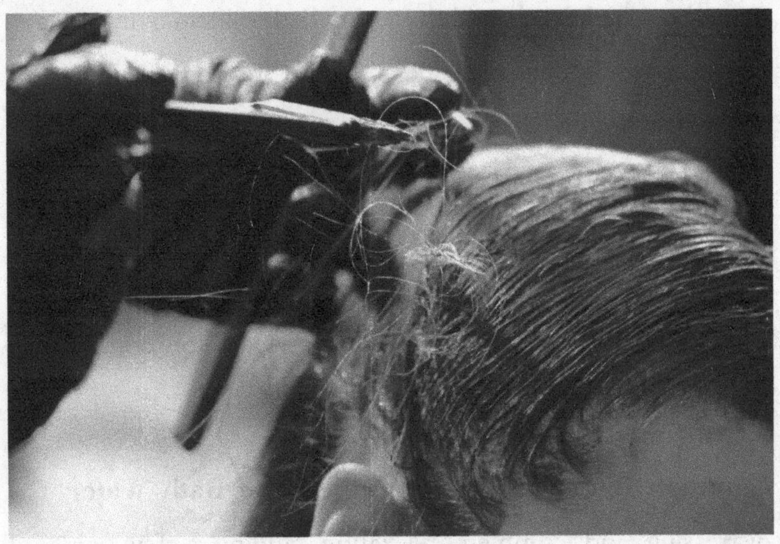

Tea as a Hair Colour: If you want black colour then try adding black tea to *henna* powder and see the difference. It helps to make the colour more intense. Black tea is an excellent temporary hair dye for those with grey hair.

Salt as Natural Cosmetics

Isn't it amazing to know that even salt can be used as a natural cosmetic? It is said that using bath salts in bath water will clear away all negative energy from your body. There are different types of salts that can be used for cosmetic purposes. Common bath salts are used for bathing purposes. There is a special bath salt called Himalayan bath salt which is said to have negative energy clearing properties. Even sea salt can be used for cosmetic purposes. Now let us see below some of the cosmetic purposes of salts.

Common Bath Salts for Adding to the Bath Water: For distressing and complete relaxation, adding a few cups of common bath salts in bath water is recommended.

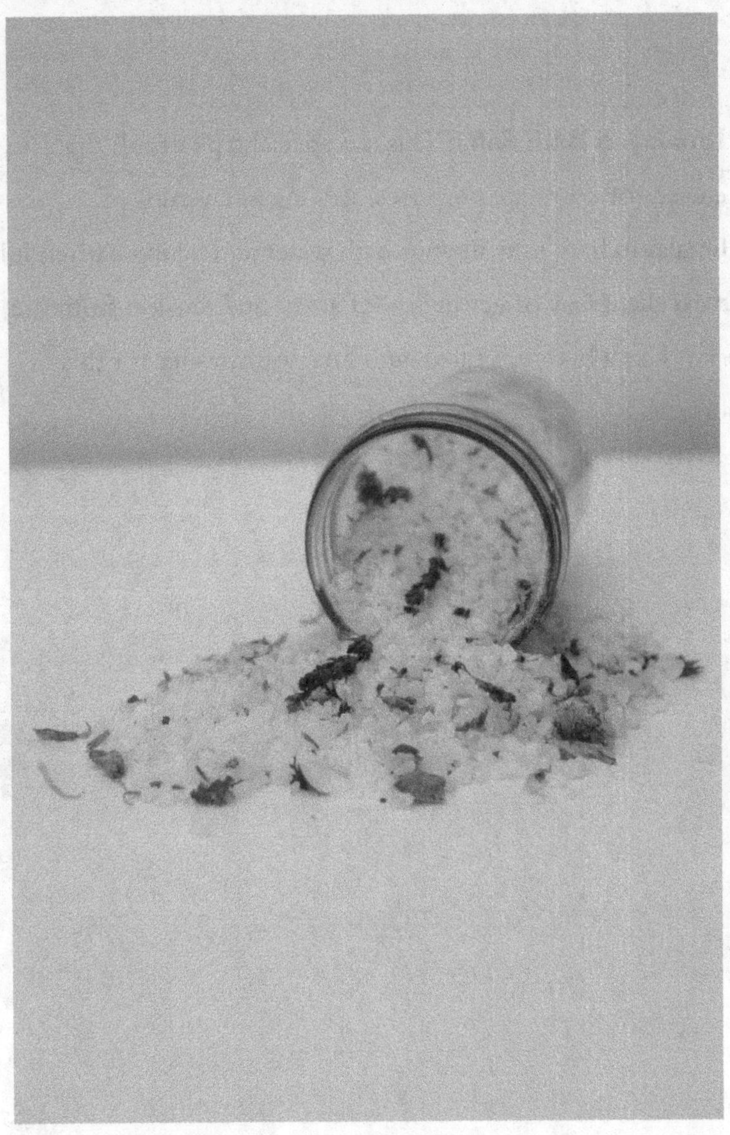

Himalayan Bath Salts: This is a special type of salt that can be used for cosmetic purposes. Adding a few cups of Himalayan bath salts in your bath water and taking bath in it is an excellent way of getting rid of stress and tension from the body. Use a bath tub filled with luke warm water for this purpose.

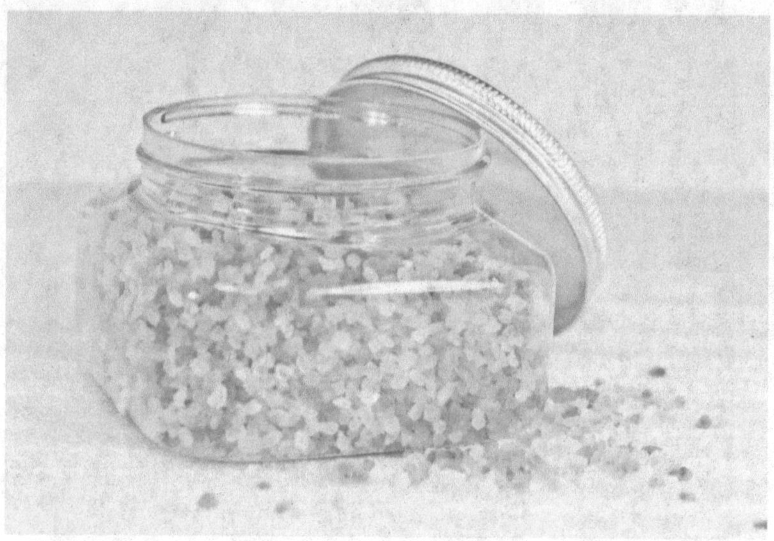

Sea Salt Facial: Sea salt-based facial is the latest trend in the beauty industry. It is said to have a deep cleansing effect on the face.

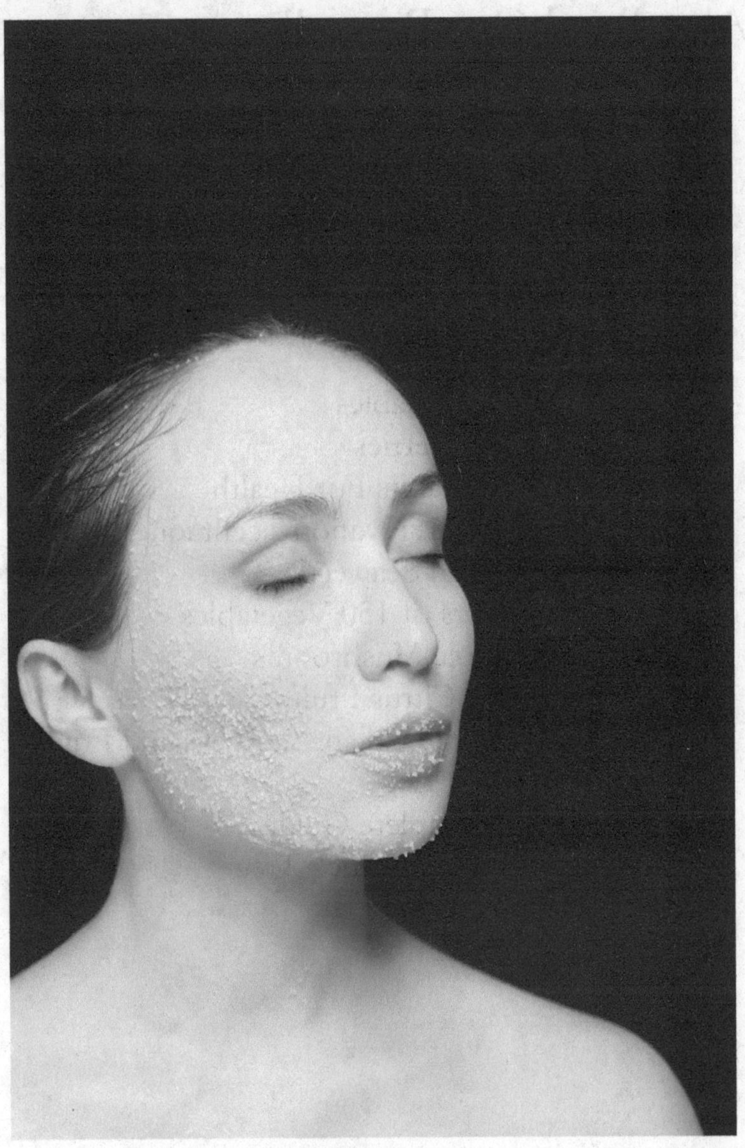

Also Read Our Bestsellers ...

1. Growing Herbs For Aromatherapy
2. Growing A Home Garden
3. Fruit Plants For Home Gardening
4. Common Medicinal Plants
5. Indoor Gardening
6. Rare Garden Plants
7. Roots as Vegetables
8. Nightshade Vegetables
9. Nutrient-Rich Berries
10. Simple Food Habits For Health
11. Simple Food Preservation Techniques
12. Mushrooms and Seaweeds
13. Health Benefits of 150 Vegetables
14. Growing Edible Mushrooms
15. Nutrient Rich Citrus Fruits
16. Mouth-Watering Indian Chutneys and Fruit Pickles
17. Tomato: A Complete Guide
18. Moringa: The Drumstick Tree
19. Curry Leaf Plant
20. Jalapeno Peppers

9 798339 069218